FOOD
IS YOUR
BEST MEDICINE

FOOD
IS YOUR
BEST MEDICINE

By HENRY G. BIELER, M.D.

VINTAGE BOOKS

A Division of Random House, New York

VINTAGE BOOKS EDITION, February 1972

Copyright © 1965 by Henry G. Bieler

All rights reserved under International and Pan-American Copyright Conventions. Published in the United States by Random House, Inc., New York, and simultaneously in Canada by Random House of Canada Limited, Toronto. Originally published by Random House, Inc., in February 1966.

Library of Congress Cataloging in Publication Data
Bieler, Henry G
  Food is your best medicine.
  1. Diet in disease. I. Title.
[RM216.B55 1973]   615′.854   72–8363
ISBN 0–394–71837–2

Manufactured in the United States of America

This book is dedicated to Frederick N. Gilbert, lawyer, humanitarian and seeker after the truth.

To The Reader

As a practicing physician for over fifty years, I have reached three basic conclusions as to the cause and cure of disease. This book is about those conclusions.

The first is that the primary cause of disease is not germs. Rather, I believe that disease is caused by a toxemia which results in cellular impairment and breakdown, thus paving the way for the multiplication and onslaught of germs.

My second conclusion is that in almost all cases the use of drugs in treating patients is harmful. Drugs often cause serious side effects, and sometimes even create new diseases. The dubious benefits they afford the patient are at best temporary. Yet the number of drugs on the market increases geometrically every year as each chemical firm develops its own variation of the compounds. The physician is indeed rare who can be completely aware of the potential danger from the side effects of all of these drugs.

My third conclusion is that disease can be cured through the proper use of correct foods. This statement may sound deceptively simple, but I have arrived at it only after intensive study of a highly complex subject: colloid and endocrine chemistry.

My conclusions are based on experimental and observational results, gathered through years of successfully treating patients. Occasionally I have resorted to the use of drugs in emergency situations, but those times have been rare. Instead, I have sought to prescribe for my patients' illnesses antidotes which Nature has placed at their disposal.

This book deals with what I consider to be the best food and the best medicine.

AN APPRECIATION

First thanks for help on this book must go to Elizabeth, who worked joyfully with me through the years.

I am also indebted to Maxine Block for her invaluable help in arranging the material and simplifying some of the professional language. She is truly remarkable, and it was a pleasure to have her editorial assistance.

Thanks should go as well to little Alana Blumer, whose criticism was always helpful.

Finally, I am deeply grateful to Robert Specht, who drew together all of our efforts.

Contents

INTRODUCTION • xiii

PART I. THE MAGNIFICENT HUMAN BODY

1 The Cure Is Worse than the Disease 3
2 Your Body: A Do-It-Yourself Repair Shop 14
3 Disease Has Many Faces 29
4 Cornerstones in My House of Health 36
5 Digestion: First Line of Defense Against Disease 54
6 The Liver: Second Line of Defense Against Disease 62
7 The Endocrine Glands: Third Line of Defense Against Disease 69
8 You—Under the Doctor's Eye 77

PART II. WHEN THE MAGNIFICENT HUMAN BODY BREAKS DOWN

9 When Disease Strikes Children 99
10 Cholesterol and the Troubled Heart 113
11 Defects in Kidneys and Blood Pressure 129
12 Your Weight: Too High or Too Low? 143
13 From Appendicitis to Women's Ailments 157

PART III.   FOOD IS YOUR BEST MEDICINE

14 Proteins Are Body Builders   177
15 Proteins Can Be Body Killers   186
16 Vegetables as Do-It-Yourself Therapy   200
17 Milk and Yeast as Food and Medicine   208
18 Salt and Stimulation vs. the Good Diet   218

INDEX • 231

Introduction

When I was a medical school student in the early days of the century, the study of nutrition was very sketchy; even today most doctors are painfully ignorant of the real advances in nutritional science. I began to suspect the close relationship between health and proper eating habits when, early in my career as an overworked young doctor, my own health broke down. I have always been a man of great curiosity and as I investigated deeply the chemistry of food along new lines, I came to the conclusion that I, personally, must give up the use of drugs and henceforth rely solely on food as my medicine. It wasn't long until (after repeated verified results) I discarded drugs in treating my patients.

My colleagues, at the time, thought I had lost my mind. But time has only strengthened my belief.

Today we are not only in the Atomic Age but also the Antibiotic Age. Unhappily, too, this is the Dark Age of Medicine—an age in which many of my colleagues, when confronted with a patient, consult a volume which rivals the Manhattan telephone directory in size. This book contains the names of thousands upon thousands of drugs used to alleviate the distressing symptoms of a host of diseased states of the body. The doctor then decides which pink or purple or baby-blue pill to prescribe for the patient.

This is not, in my opinion, the practice of medicine.

Far too many of these new "miracle" drugs are introduced with fanfare and then revealed as lethal in character, to be silently discarded for newer and more powerful drugs, which allegedly cure all the ills to which the flesh is heir.

I discarded drugs partly because I began to re-examine an old, old 'medical truism—that nature does the real healing, utilizing the natural defenses of the body. Under the proper conditions nature, if given the opportunity, is always the greatest healer. It is the physician's role to assist in this healing—to co-operate with nature's forces; to play a supporting role instead of star of the show. Nature does not follow Madison Avenue's "Feel Better Faster" but takes her time, slowly, as a tree grows, a little more each day. Nature never rushes to get a sick man or beast on his feet; she also demands a slow and steady convalescence. Sick animals rest or sleep and refuse all food until nature has healed them.

Isn't it proper, then, to expect that nature can do the same thing for the sick human if only she is given the opportunity?

Because I believe this so deeply, I have been in disagreement with doctors who stuff the sick, exhausted man with powerful toxic drugs and then are forced to use other drugs to "remedy the remedy," as it were. Instead I "fast" the patient on simple vegetable broths or diluted fruit juices in order to give the exhausted body organs an opportunity to discharge their waste products and heal themselves.

Call me "controversial" if you will; I have taken the revered Louis Pasteur off his pedestal. Years of laboratory observation and experimentation have taught me that germs do not cause disease. Germs are merely a concomitant of disease, present in every sick individual but able to multiply in a sick person because of disturbed function.

Every new concept developed in medical science points the way to a new area awaiting further exploration. Discarding both the use of drugs and the germ theory of disease opened the way for me to explore new methods of eliminating the stagnating waste products from the body. Briefly stated, my position is: improper foods cause disease; proper foods cure disease. In upholding this thesis, I have been in disagreement, at times sharp, with organized orthodox medicine.

While seeking additional methods to aid in this elimination of toxins, I began a study along original lines, here and in Europe, of just how I could use the endocrine glands, particularly the liver, adrenal, thyroid and pituitary glands. From there, my medical curiosity led me to a study of the harm done to the body by various stimulating foods and non-foods, such as salt.

The average American predilection for doughnuts and coffee, hot dogs with mustard, ice cream, fried meat, French-fried potatoes, pie à la mode, together with between-meal sweetened cola drinks, candy bars and coffee breaks, synthetic vitamins and aspirin cannot make for health. And they cannot make for a pure cholesterol. Long before cholesterol became a household word I was interested in its role in the body. Here you will find a unique approach to the cholesterol problem and also how to build a pure cholesterol which wears well in the arteries.

In these pages you will discover which foods are helpful and which harmful and how the body reacts to both in health and in illness. You will notice that, though there are suggestions about eating or not eating (for when *not* to eat is often more important than what to eat), there is no cure-all diet suggested for whatever ails you.

As a child of four back in Cincinnati, Ohio, I announced to my parents one day that I wanted to be a doctor. For over fifty years now I have been a doctor—not a specialist, merely a general practitioner. I have treated motion picture stars and coal miners; politicians and professional men; farmers and Pasadena society dowagers; I have brought thousands of healthy babies into the world, including my own children and grandchildren. A decade ago, I thought I might retire and devote myself to my hobbies—music, reading, sculpture, mountain climbing and wild animal study—so I closed my Pasadena office and built a glass-walled house on a sea cliff, high above the sun-warmed Pacific. But patients from near and far (even from abroad) sought me out in a steady stream seven days a week, to learn how proper food, individually selected for their particular ills, will cure them. If I have helped them back to health, I am well rewarded, for in the process I have become not only a counselor but a friend.

Henry G. Bieler, M.D.
Capistrano Beach, 1965

PART I

THE MAGNIFICENT HUMAN BODY

1

The Cure Is Worse than the Disease

> To live by medicine is to live horribly.
> —CARL LINNAEUS (1707–1778)
>
> Eighteen times in every second a prescription is filled
> by a white-coated pharmacist at one of the fifty-six
> thousand drugstores in the United States. The stag-
> gering cost of these pink, violet, yellow, white
> and green tablets, capsules, lozenges, and ampules
> amounts to $3 billion a year.
> —MARGUERITE CLARK, MEDICINE TODAY, 1960

Twenty-five hundred years ago on the island of Cos in classical
Greece a bearded physician-teacher, Hippocrates, sat in the shade
of an Oriental plane tree on a lovely hillside and admonished his
wide-eyed circle of medical students in one of his most pithy and
precise aphorisms: "Thy food shall be thy remedy."

No one, to date, has more eloquently given us a way of life.

The medical profession insists it strives to emulate the Father of
All Physicians and, indeed, is required, before licensing, to take
the Hippocratic Oath, one of the most sublime declamations for
lofty ethical standards ever penned. Yet today there are thousands
of dedicated bacteriologists, pharmaceutical researchers and chemists sitting in gleaming white laboratories in every major city

throughout the world, busily turning out synthetic, if highly touted, magic panaceas for every known ailment. Unlike that of the venerable Hippocrates, their battle cry appears to be: "Thy remedy shall be our newly invented remedy."

Yet despite the advances in technological knowledge and the millions spent on medical research programs, mankind sickens and dies; hospitals and mental institutions are filled to overflowing with the diseased and the hopeless. Here in our own country—where the greatest abundance of foodstuffs and the highest living standards in history are to be found—a truly radiantly healthy person is as rare as a pearl in a barrel of oysters. And although extremely low standards of physical fitness were used, approximately 40 percent of America's young men were judged unfit for military service in World War II. Three times during the last decade military physical-fitness requirements were lowered. So that while we are the most wealthy country in the world, we are also, comparatively, one of the least healthy.

Why?

What of the future?

Our forecasts for the continued increase in the incidence of cancer, high blood pressure, heart disease—in fact, all the degenerative diseases—are most dismal.

To be sure, new drugs and techniques are waging battle against these great killers. And some succeed. "More often," admits Furness Thompson, vice-president of a large drug laboratory, "failure is our most important product." While it is true that no medicine is innocent, one cause of grave concern is the untoward reactions these sometimes dangerously potent drugs may cause—reactions which may extend far into the future. Another serious adverse result of the use of certain drugs is the possibility of addiction. And when the layman goes in for self-medication, using drugs prescribed for others, the results may become truly catastrophic.

Patients storm doctors' offices, begging for a "quick cure" with a "miracle drug" they've just read about in their newspapers, only to discover—in increasing numbers—side effects so serious that presently they have *additional* disorders in urgent need of treatment. So the help they seek is often outweighed by the tragic damage to the body. And although millions are spent for clinical testing the study of the action and effects of these extremely hazardous drugs is still in its infancy. One day a new drug is hailed with typical Hollywood fanfare, as a potential life saver; six months later it is silently withdrawn as a lethal weapon. If patients hounding doctors for a newly available miracle drug would only realize that a sound evaluation of a drug takes months and even years of painstaking work, would they be so anxious to serve as guinea pigs?

Unhappily, anxiety-ridden Americans, following the warning voices of televised drug commercials and newspaper ads, consider health something that can be purchased in a bottle at the drugstore; they forget, or never knew, that health can be found only by obeying the clear-cut laws of nature.

Examples are numerous. Everyone recalls the dramatic headlines, following the too careless use of the European tranquilizer Thalidomide; more shocking was the tragic aftermath of armless and legless babies born to women who took the drug during the early months of pregnancy.

And yet, why did so many European and American women use Thalidomide? Why did many pregnant women offer it to friends who were expecting? Because it brought relief from natural symptoms. When nature starts a pregnancy, she makes strenuous efforts to eliminate all the old accumulated toxic matter in the woman's body in order to have a cleaner chemical field for the gestation of the fetus. The womb suddenly is transformed from an organ through which vicarious elimination of toxins can take place into a non-menstruating organ which must act as a receptacle for the developing child.

My studies have shown that to facilitate the cleansing process, the mother's body throws out a great deal of its background toxemia through the liver as an irritating bile. As this is eliminated it causes all the side reactions which may be classified under the heading "toxemia of pregnancy": nausea, vomiting, fatigue, nervousness, indigestion, headache. Many afflicted women gulped Thalidomide as a miraculous cure for their distress. How tragic that the penalty for numbing the distressing symptoms of early pregnancy should have resulted in such catastrophe!

When a fad develops for a new drug, it can cause extensive damage; the tranquilizers and corticoids are prime examples. Not so well known was the great fad of cod liver oil therapy, now happily on the wane. One cannot help but wonder how many new diseases have been created en route by the barrels and barrels of fish oil for the cure and prevention of rickets. The livers of the dolphin, the cod, the halibut and the shark have been duly processed, clarified, bleached, boiled and refined until they have lost all possible resemblance to their original state.

Although I have delivered thousands of babies over the years (including my own children and grandchildren), I have never used cod liver oil. The babies thrived on a diet of raw milk and raw sugar, with fruits and vegetables added after six months.

The cod liver oil theory was knocked flat by the experiments and observations of Dr. Francis F. Pottenger, Jr. (I will have more to say about his monumental work in another connection.) Dr. Pottenger, in proving that a diet of cooked meat was totally inadequate for carnivorous animals, found that his experimental cats quickly developed rickets. Cod liver oil (the classic remedy) was then administered in increasing doses until it thoroughly purged the sick cats. Unhappily, the rickets remained and a new complication appeared: disturbed digestions. For cod liver oil not only upsets the chemistry of digestion and of the liver but it also causes injury or degeneration to other important organs of the body, especially the thyroid gland, the heart and liver. Yet how many well-meaning mothers are still cramming this evil-tasting oil into their babies' throats today.

Experiments confirming the harmful effects of drugs, from slight to sinister, are legion. Yet public interest in new drugs just off the laboratory assembly line is so phenomenal that newspapers and magazines make them front-page news. After amazing reports of an experimental "miracle" drug (written in a *bang-bang!* style) appear in a weekly news magazine, doctors may be certain that next morning patients will storm in demanding it.

One *bang-bang!* drug is the celebrated penicillin. As everyone knows, penicillin is a most powerful and valuable agent for the treatment of staphyloccocal and other infections in man. But given indiscriminately for fevers and infections of the respiratory tract, it may have allergic and toxic qualities which are highly dangerous. Just recently, the Los Angeles *Times* carried the report of a twenty-two-year-old mother who died twenty minutes after she was given a penicillin shot as a precautionary measure to fend off an oncoming cold. She suffered a fatal reaction, despite having experienced no ill effect from "numerous injections" of the drug in the past.

One of the great dangers of the ever lengthening list of antibiotics arises when physicians use them too freely. Some people become very sensitive to antibiotics after they have been given them too many times. The reason for this is that the large molecules in antibiotics readily form antigens with proteins. When this happens, antibodies are formed in the body. If, then, another injection of penicillin is given, disaster arises when it comes in contact with the antibodies within the cells. People who become sensitive also become allergic to the drug. This allergy may show merely as a mild skin rash in some cases; in others it may mean sudden death as a result of anaphylactic shock. Medical literature lists well over a hundred deaths following injections of penicillin. One of the cases described was that of a woman who sprained a toe: as she had for all sorts of minor illnesses in the past, she gratefully accepted a penicillin injection; but she did not survive her visit to the doctor's office.

From my own files I know of two cases in which physicians used penicillin with unhappy results. A woman of thirty-six, in apparent good health, suffered from a cold and headache. Penicillin was given, although the symptoms were mild and there was no fever. The injection increased the headache. The following day the injection was repeated. This increased the headache enormously. As a result of overstimulation, the pituitary gland increased in size and pressed against the delicate optic nerves. Total blindness followed, from which the patient has never recovered. Thus, pressure blindness resulted from excessive swelling of the pituitary gland brought on by penicillin, a toxic drug. It is, in fact, so toxic that it is thrown out by the kidneys just a few seconds after it is injected, despite the scientific efforts of the pharmacologists to prevent its rapid elimination. Penicillin often accomplishes truly miraculous results by whipping the endocrine glands into hyperactivity. But in the case cited above—*overstimulation* of the pituitary gland—it brought a tragic result.

In the second case a young couple, both in good physical condition, planned their marriage. Just before the wedding the bride contracted a slight cold. Her doctor gave her an injection of penicillin. An acute vaginitis followed (redness, swelling and pain) which lasted for several years, precluding any sex life.

The chief therapeutic value of penicillin, I have found, lies in its ability to whip the endocrine glands to a higher tempo. The adrenals are usually the first to react. If they are strong and able, a shower of their secretion is let loose in the blood. The intense superoxidation that results raises the resistance, so that fevers, pains and other disturbing complications magically disappear. *But after each glandular whipping the energy of the adrenals is weakened.* And if the therapy is continued, they finally become exhausted.

"Defects may arise in the humors [fluids] of our bodies in any place, following the unnatural cure," said a wise old teacher of medicine at the University of Leyden, Hermann Boerhaave. Except that he was born in 1668, Boerhaave might well have been speaking of the reactions, from mild to severe, which sometimes follow the use of penicillin. For the relief or cure of these reactions pharmacologists have developed another drug. Here we have the classical example of one devil chasing out another! It is frightening to consider how much subsequent harm may result from bottling up two irritants in the unsuspecting human body. Such a thought is followed by another: all drugs which are introduced into the body are likely to have bad as well as good effects. Isn't it sensible, therefore, to restrict their use as much as possible? One area in which restriction of wonder drugs, particularly penicillin, is strongly urged is the ordinary head cold. *Penicillin has no curative effects on the common cold.* Yet untold millions of adults and children have been jabbed with useless shots of the drug while suffering from a cold. The body then has two enemies to expel: the cold and the toxic drug. If this were the only evil effect of the misuse of penicillin, it would not be too harmful. There is, in addition, the menace of adverse drug reaction, way beyond what meets the physician's eye, in damage to liver or eyes or kidneys or blood system. There may be damage which does not show up until years later. And finally, saddest of all, are the *many deaths every year* directly due to sensitivity to penicillin. It is believed by reputable scientists that in the course of a lifetime one person in every ten in this country may, because of contact with foods and cosmetics and drugs containing penicillin, become sensitized to it and not ever be able to use it again. The loss of the usefulness of penicillin would be a major catastrophe. Shouldn't we then take this powerful drug out of circulation when it comes to treating such simple conditions as the common cold? And shouldn't the American people rid themselves of the currently held *misinformation* that antibiotics are cure-alls? And this goes too for the prevalent fad of stuffing oneself with synthetic vitamins, as if these pills could rejuvenate mankind. *Instead, they line the bulging pockets of the pharmaceutical houses.*

The physician's office has become a repository for a mountain of drugs—free samples, distributed by almost twenty thousand "detail men" or professional representatives, known earlier as "drug peddlers." A doctor's office, it may be argued, is not the place to investigate the efficacy of a new drug: that should have been done long before the physician passes them out to his patients. Because these drugs are distributed as a free promotion by drug companies, Americans are being subjected to potent drugs with adverse reactions on a scale unprecedented in history. It is not too much to expect that when an individual takes a new drug he deserves to know whether he is serving as an involuntary guinea pig. This right was abused in the Thalidomide tragedy.

While it is true that drugs promising cures proliferate like rabbits, it is also true that drug making is no modern phenomenon. From the beginning of time man has searched for the potent elixir which would absolve him of his sins while allowing him to continue committing them.

Man has been called "an ingenious assembly of portable plumbing." And down that "plumbing" through the ages he has poured concoctions of powdered scorpions and bats' ears and ergot of rye and powdered opium mixed with ipecac and hensbane, dogsbane and ratsbane and deadly nightshade as well as thousands of more ordinary cure-alls. We may feel that we're living in a time of "drug hypnosis," but it was a half century before Christ when Publius Syrus sagely observed, "There are some remedies worse than the disease." Variations of this cynical remark have been made by both patients and physicians since—and very likely long before his time.

Do doctors take their own medicines? Happily, not too many do, even though a now rare synonym for doctor is "mediciner." Sir William Osler, one of the most brilliant physicians of recent times, became ill in Cannes at the turn of the century. A local physician gave him a pill containing compound of mercury, then heralded as a magic cure for many illnesses. Next morning, the pill was still on Osler's night table.

"That was a peculiar pill," Osler remarked before he dropped it in the wastebasket. It was also used as a specific cure for syphilis, until it was discovered that many of the "late tertiaries" of that disease were really caused by mercury poisoning. "The desire to take medicine is perhaps the greatest feature which distinguishes man from animals," observed Osler. "The young physician starts life with twenty drugs for each disease and the old physician ends life with one drug for twenty diseases."

I confess that I, too, as an eager medical school graduate (and for some years afterwards) stuffed my patients with pills, potions and panaceas before I, like Macbeth, decided to "Throw physic to the dogs; I'll none of it." And found that dogs—smart creatures they—merely sniffed at them and trotted away.

How I personally emerged from this state of "drug hypnosis," how and why I returned to natural processes and came to discard drugs in favor of food as the best medicine, is a long story which I will discuss in these pages, in addition to making a good many observations on the cause and cure of disease. For the moment, let it suffice to say that at one point in my career, instead of looking forward to the next miracle drug to emerge from the test tube, I began to wonder if the time hadn't come to rediscover some ancient truths, some amazingly sharp insights into medicine as practiced by some of the world's greatest physicians of the past.

Recently, while browsing through some fairly new medical books, I came across one in which Oliver Wendell Holmes was mentioned in apologetic tones as the benign old gentleman who wrote "The Chambered Nautilus," even though he made one of the most penetrating studies in the history of medicine, on the causes of various fevers. Dr. Holmes has been hailed as "the most successful combination the world has ever seen, of physician and man of letters." One of his maxims, although so often quoted that it has lost its pungency, is nevertheless more applicable today than when he wrote it a hundred years ago:

> I firmly believe if the whole *materia medica* as now used could be sunk to the bottom of the sea, it would be all the better for mankind—and all the worse for the fishes.

It was precisely because of the poor, drugged "human fishes" that throughout the centuries many men of medicine have pointed to the importance of food and to the relative incompetence of drugs when considering health and disease. The greatest physicians have used the fewest and simplest of drugs, because they were fully aware of the role of nature in health; they knew that all the forces of nature in man, beast and the plant world are dedicated to obtaining and keeping a perfect state of health. They knew that many diseases are "self-limited," that is, they cure themselves whether you do anything or nothing for them.

We see this in Hippocrates' basic precept that "Nature heals; the physician is only nature's assistant." And when the Father of Clinical Medicine forsook potent and poisonous drugs in favor of the profoundly simple and sane belief in the healing power of nature, assisted by good food, fresh air, rest, recreation, sleep, change of climate and physiotherapy, he inaugurated the Golden Age of Greek medicine.

As I studied medical history, I became more and more convinced that drugs are not the path to restoration of health. What was it that made the reputation of Thomas Sydenham, the pioneer English physician of the seventeenth century? I tend to think it was a blend of common sense and genius which gained for him the title of the "English Hippocrates" and which caused the revered Boerhaave of Leyden to uncover his head whenever Sydenham's name was mentioned. (Boerhaave, himself, was no upstart. Once he received a letter from a doctor in China, merely addressed "To the most famous physician in Europe.") Sydenham used the simplest of remedies when he *knew* what was wrong with the patient; when he *didn't know*, he observed the patient closely and used no remedies at all. He dared to "order fresh air for small pox patients and riding on horseback for consumptives, in place of the smothering system and the noxious and often loathsome rubbish of the established schools."

Fresh air was a new therapy in Sydenham's day. And today a search for pure air, pure raw milk, pure water, natural, unprocessed, unpreserved foods, unsprayed vegetables, nourishing whole-grain bread is too simple, too unpretentious to be extolled as a "new" therapy in treating disease.

Today, too, the physician is inclined to discount the natural wisdom of the body itself; to forget that the body has two small bean-shaped master chemists of its own: the kidneys, whose tasks are more complex than any electronic computer conceived by man. Instead, a growing number of physicians are more likely to get writers' cramp making out prescriptions for patients who are demanding them, the while forgetting the story of the physician who handed a prescription to a patient, saying: "Here, have this filled quickly, while it is still a remedy."

Away back in the year 1855 (drugs were even then the chief remedy for disease), the following notice was posted by the Massachusetts Medical Society:

The Treasurer announced that he had received the sum of one hundred dollars from a member of the Society for a prize . . . on the following theme: "We would regard every approach toward the rational and successful prevention and management of a disease, without the necessity of drugs, to be an advance in favor of humanity and scientific medicine."

What I hope to do in this book is show you that both "prevention and management" of disease may be obtained without drugs. I have done it more times than I am able to count. Although my solution to this problem may come too late to be rewarded by that famous posted prize, I hope it will still be in time to do much good.

2
Your Body: A Do-It-Yourself Repair Shop

> The aim of medicine is to prevent disease and pro-
> long life; the ideal of medicine is to eliminate the
> need of a physician.
>
> —WILLIAM J. MAYO, M.D.

The human body is an incomparable instrument, a marvelous
mechanism, truly breathtaking in its intricacy. To the followers of
Hippocrates and Galen, that medical giant of the Middle Ages, it
is a fascinating, if never-ending study—before which the most
learned scientist stands in reverent awe. He stands in awe, too, of
the body's amazing capacity to repair its own injuries and to heal
its illnesses.

We have much to learn about the body, but what we already
know shows us that it operates in a manner we can understand.
What we cannot understand is the problem of *why* man's magnificently engineered body should be riddled with disease. Dr. Albert V. Szent-Györgyi, the distinguished Hungarian biochemist
who was awarded a Nobel Prize in 1937 for identifying Vitamin C,
has beautifully expressed this enigma:

> The general problem of health and disease which has occupied
> my mind very much for my whole scientific career is dominated
> by two big contradictory impressions. As a medical student, I

learned about those *thousand diseases* humanity is suffering from. . . . Since then, as a biochemist, I am living in silent admiration of the wonderful precision, adaptability and perfection of our body. Medicine taught me the shocking imperfection, biochemistry the wonderful perfection, and I have wondered where the contradiction lies. Anything that Nature produces seems to be perfect. Should, then, man be the only imperfect creature kept alive in the face of all his imperfections only by means created by his own mind? *If not, where do all these ailments come from; how must we understand them?* This is the great fundamental problem of medicine, the great fundamental problem of Health and Disease, and we must try to answer these problems and try to advance from the description of the single diseases to *some more general conception of health and disease;* such a concept might help us in our efforts to lead humanity towards a period of better health and greater happiness.

When, as a busy, hard-working physician shortly after World War I, my own health deteriorated, I became more interested than ever in the cause of disease. At first I was too engrossed in my practice to note how I felt; finally I had to take time to look into my own condition. Doctors do not make good patients; they know too much and it is difficult for them (or anyone) to adjust to the idea of illness in themselves. We all resist the unpleasant. But when a "sick" doctor finally gets busy with his own maladies, his technical knowledge of how disease operates makes it easier for him to continue on a course of treatment.

Plato said that no physician could treat a disease really well until he has had it himself. I don't completely agree, but I do know that one of the most valuable lessons I learned from this unhappy period was how much a previously healthy physician gains from his experience when illness strikes.

I was an orthodox general practitioner and naturally I tried all that orthodox medicine had to offer. To my dismay, I wasn't relieved in any way. I had asthma and I had kidney trouble; I was also grossly overweight.

Fortunately, I met a doctor who was well versed in chemical pathology and whose revolutionary theories on the cause and cure of disease fired my imagination. We discussed my illness in such an illuminating manner that within five minutes I knew the path I had to follow. Before I met him I did not know that nutritional problems will never respond to stuffing oneself with medicine, a course I'd been following. I plunged into concentrated study and soon I was ready to discard my dietary errors as well as the medicines I was taking. Released from the overstimulation of both improper foods and harmful medicines, my infirmities disappeared and have never returned; my weight dropped from 210 to 137, then rose to 155. Thereafter it remained stationary, which for my height and bone structure I consider perfect.

What, exactly, was the regime I followed? What magical foods had brought about this restoration of my health? Whenever I have mentioned my own experiences to a patient, I have been asked these questions. Possibly you too are asking them. Yet there is nothing to be gained by mere recital, because every individual, medically speaking, is an island unlike any other. He requires a program custom-tailored to his unique needs. And that is why mail-order diagnosis and treatment can result only in harm. Doctors, who should know better, especially those who envy my energy and buoyant health, frequently ask me about my personal regime. I cannot tell you exactly what to eat but I plan to give you general rules for diet in combating or preventing disease—rules which you may profitably apply in your individual case. For proper food is not just for the health faddist but is, when you are aware of the facts, truly a way of life.

As for myself, the results, achieved merely through dietary reform, appeared well nigh magical to an orthodox practitioner of medicine of a half century ago. My interest in diet as a therapeutic measure was not shared by many doctors following World War I. It was a time when only cultists on the fringe of medicine believed that overstimulating foods and medicines, excesses of sugar and starches, condiments, alcohol and tobacco could possibly play roles in bringing disease to a healthy body. The average doctor, busy handing out prescriptions, had forgotten the words of Peter Mere Latham (b. 1789): "In regard to such diseases, especially, as are engendered by defective nutrition, we know it to be a matter of experience, that they are generally capable of being speedily and effectually cured by an improved diet." Such truths as these contributed by early medical men are still applicable today, even though the last fifty years have produced tremendous advances in our scientific knowledge.

So I renewed my acquaintance with Dr. Latham and others; I directed my attention to the cure of disease from the angle of the chemistry of endocrinology, food chemistry and the whole field of the chemistry of metabolism. I realized that you cannot use the whip of stimulant (improper food and medicines) on the back of a drugged, exhausted and ill individual without serious results. And through the years, I added to my knowledge whenever and wherever I could. Now, after fifty years of experience, I still consider myself a student, because the medical scene changes constantly and I have never lost my insatiable curiosity in the role nutrition plays in health—the same interest which animated me when my own health broke down.

Before I began my studies in nutrition and the chemistry of the endocrine system, my own eating habits had been atrocious, judged by what is common knowledge today. For instance, while waiting for my dinner, I was in the habit of shaking a little salt in the palm of my hand and licking it until the meal was served. Without tasting the food my wife placed before me, I automatically reached for the salt cellar. Salt made me feel good; I employed it as a means of stimulation, just as others enjoy coffee, tobacco or alcohol—none of which I used. I was a heavy eater, a trencherman who liked all the starches. Lunch and dinner were incomplete without a heavy dessert and a quart of milk was just an incidental in the meal.

I wasn't aware that my eating habits were harmful; I ate what I liked and would have considered any advice to change as sheer nonsense. From cradle to coffin, food is a major concern and there-fore not easily tampered with. Any obese person, engaged in a struggle to lose weight, knows this only too well. The tenacity of food habits, good or bad, was brought to me strongly when I read in the Los Angeles *Times* an interview given by Miss Edith Jones, president of the American Dietetic Association, an organization of sixteen thousand dietitians. Miss Jones, a native of Alabama, hasn't lost her taste for Southern cooking: "I still like my snap beans boiled three hours," she admitted. "I grew up with them cooked that way. Just don't pour off the water they're cooked in. But I don't recommend this as an ideal way to cook beans in a hospital." Miss Jones knows what happens to enzymes and vitamins during three hours of boiling, but she's not about to change her lifelong habit.

I, however, was ready and willing to make a change when illness came. And at the time when I radically revised my method of eating and began, as a consequence, to lose considerable weight on my new diet, I recall that my orthodox medical colleagues eyed me warily, and I overheard whispers: "Bieler is starving himself to death. He's going crazy." And a year or so later when, after much research, I stopped using medicines entirely in my practice because I obtained better results through the chemistry of food and the chemistry of the glands—a more lasting effect and one less detri-mental in the long run—my friends shook their collective heads in wonder.

They considered me a renegade from established practices of dosing patients with medicines; they expected me to jump back on their bandwagon if I wanted to cure patients. Really, there is no special medicine which is a specific (or remedy) for any *chronic* disease. Even the miracle drugs, shamefully overadvertised, cannot perform this miracle. *For the truth is that 80 to 85 percent of all types of human ailments are self-limited, that is, they run their course and the individual recovers.* Whether the drugs he takes help or not is often a matter of argument among members of the medi-cal profession. I choose to believe that most drugs are unnecessary or even detrimental. I choose to believe, too, that misguided enthusiasts among the medical profession are "overtreating" patients. And our medical journals, with commendable honesty, are today discussing "*iatrogenic*" or "physician-generated" disease.

To return to the role of nutrition in disease, I would like to point out that the study of nutrition as a separate science is barely forty years old. As I look back on my medical school days I realize (as have many other doctors who left medical school more recently) that I had learned little of value about dietetics. It was scarcely considered a part of the medical curriculum in the early days of the century. Nor is there much change today. And this in the face of Hippocrates' belief that the physician should "Leave thy drugs in the chemist's pot if thou can'st heal the patient with food."

So it is understandable that if you dare mention dietetics to the orthodox medical man as a possible cure for disease, he is likely to listen with a good deal of skepticism. If you suggest that diet may play a role in arthritis, he will throw up his hands in horror.

Yet my files show that 95 percent of my patients who were badly crippled by arthritis and suffering constant pain, have been either freed of both or left with a small amount of residual pain and stiffness. In general, my treatment for arthritis is prolonged, but in a small number of cases all the pain left the joints within two weeks of beginning treatment. Here is one case from my files: A fifty-five-year-old woman attempted to commit suicide because of extreme depression. On her first visit she complained of heart palpitation and inability to sleep; her blood pressure was 160/100; her urine was extremely acid; her knees, ankles and feet were so swollen, feverish and painful that she said she could hardly get up and down street curbs. She also complained of stiffness and pain in her hands, left hip and shoulder. "I'm headed in a direct path to a wheel chair," she confessed.

She was in the habit of drinking about twelve cups of coffee a day, smoked a great deal, ate much meat, starches, canned fruit and sweets and used aspirin to relieve pain. On this diet it followed that she was overweight.

"I'm willing to give you a complete year of my life to see if you can make me well," she declared dramatically.

"It will probably take much longer than that," I warned her. "Your joints didn't stiffen in a day; the toxic saturation of your body has been years in developing. Also, you've been palliating your symptoms with drugs and, together with improper food, that has brought you to your present physical and mental condition."

I convinced her to give up all drugs, smoking, coffee and meat for her particular case, although I do permit some patients to eat meat and drink weak tea or coffee. She was given calcium capsules as her only medication and the following foods: upon arising, one cake of yeast dissolved in warm water; for breakfast, a vegetable soup of string beans and zucchini; mid-morning, four ounces of raw milk; for lunch, cooked celery, more vegetable soup, one slice of bread and lettuce salad without dressing; mid-afternoon, fruit or fruit juice diluted with water; dinner, one package of frozen or ten ounces fresh cut green beans, lightly cooked including the liquid from the pan and a head of lettuce; before retiring, another yeast cake in water.

Three years later her weight had gone down to normal; her blood pressure was 120/100; her depression had left completely; she slept well and was able to work hard. "It seems like a miracle to be free of arthritis," she reported. "There is not a single twinge of pain any more and no swelling any place. I'm feeling happier than I ever have and I never get tired of my diet, although it was awfully hard to get used to it at first. Sometimes, for short periods, I went off of my diet because I'd have a yearning for sweets and meat. Strangely enough, they didn't taste nearly as good as I thought. And when I saw how much better I felt without them, I always returned gladly to my diet for I had a dogged determination to stay out of that wheel chair. My whole body feels better, my skin has improved and everyone tells me how much better I look."

It is true that most doctors would consider such a case history too fantastic to be believed. And if you are brave enough, in talking to a doctor, to link diet with that emotionally charged disease, cancer, you are frequently left talking to the wind. Yet Dr. Frederick Hoffman, for many years chief statistician of the Prudential Life Insurance Company, is the author of a dictionary-sized book on cancer and diet written after he had made exhaustive studies all over the world. Dr. Hoffman concludes: "I am fully convinced that profound dietary influences in cancer are to be looked upon as a causative factor." Still, it is heresy to mention diet and cancer in the same sentence or diet and any disease which the medical profession believes can only be "cured" through a pill or an injection. We are so concerned with synthesizing chemicals which will cure that we have lost sight of the fact that these same chemicals have been lodged in our foods for many thousands of years.

Throughout the years I have been able to observe the close relationship of diet and disease in my own patients. I recall the first tumor case I treated by diet, many, many years ago. I must confess I knew practically nothing about the relationship between the two when a farmer's wife came to my office. Above her collar bone, she had a fibroid tumor about the size of a turkey egg (and almost as firm) covered with a post-operative scar.

"The surgeon could not remove it after he began to operate," she explained, "because it was so deeply buried in the nerves and blood vessels. I've heard that you use diet as a cure and I read in a magazine that tumors could be reduced by following the correct diet. Can you help me?"

"I'm not certain that I know how to proceed," I told her. Upon examination of her urine, I found a tremendous excess of sulphur proteins. When I asked her what she had been eating, she explained that she and her husband owned a turkey ranch and that before the tumor developed she had been eating turkey three times a day for a good many months because they had been unable to sell their turkeys. Although I confessed that I did not know what treatment to follow, I suggested that we proceed to remove all the sulphur from her diet and then increase its alkaline side through the use of vegetables and fruits. She immediately omitted the sulphur-rich vegetables of the cabbage family and others and, of course, animal and seafood proteins which are also rich in sulphur.

After six months on this rigid sulphur-free diet we were delighted to find the tumor half as large as it had been. And after one year it had disappeared entirely. I am by nature a cautious soul and it was only then that I began to think there must be something in this form of therapy after all. Here was a rock-hard, inoperable tumor. And yet it was gradually reabsorbed and eliminated by lowering the sulphur content of the blood. The patient remained on an animal-protein-free diet for two years, then she added rare beef or lamb and a small amount of milk while continuing with generous helpings of all the sulphur-free vegetables and fruits.

Twenty-seven years later, a famous and glamorous movie star came to me with a grapefruit-sized fibroid tumor of the womb. She had been advised by a well-known gynecologist at the Massachusetts General Hospital that surgical removal was necessary. When she came to me instead, I prescribed a simple diet that included cooked cereals for breakfast, plain salads for lunch, and cooked non-starchy vegetables for dinner. Animal protein was completely eliminated. Some time later she tape-recorded the following and sent it to me:

At the same time I started on your diet I went into one of the most rugged periods of my life. I had started on my own program in television and I worked every day, hours and hours and hours of physical work. I had six months of that. Then I came out to California and made a most successful movie. Mind you, I was still on string beans and zucchini while traveling, often cooked over a little burner in a bathroom. My work schedule was very tight. I used to keep a piece of bread and butter in my pocket or maybe a banana. The movie took twelve weeks to make. Then I took a trip for the studio, visiting thirty-three cities. I wore out four maids, and my secretary needed some alcohol to bolster her up at the end of the day. After the first tour I made another one, so in all I spent a year doing nothing but traveling—a different city every other day. There were no free weekends during this work.

All of a sudden, two and a half years had passed and I found myself up in Boston, Mass. I had realized, by feeling my tummy in the morning, that the hard lump had disappeared.

I had a real sense of great health and I went to see the doctor who had previously examined me. He was furious that he had never heard from me since the first examination and was sure that he was going to find a mess confronting him. I watched his face while he was examining me and I must say that he was a baffled doctor. He went and got the examination card to see exactly whether there had been such a tumor, the size of a grapefruit. When he came back I said: "It's gone, isn't it doctor?" He said it was gone, all right, but he still couldn't believe it. Then I said: "Don't you want to know how or why? I've been on a non-protein diet—no animal protein at all." "Well," he said, throwing his head back and laughing, "I think that's ridiculous." Then he said that it would have gone anyway. I said: "Yes, I know, about a year and a half ago, by your knife." I got up and dressed. I was grinning when I left his office as I asked him whether he didn't think Nature was wonderful.

Since then, among my patients there have been many cases of fibroid tumors elsewhere in the body which have been banished merely by changes in the diet. Seems remarkable, doesn't it? Other patients, with various afflictions, do not have the stamina to remain on the rigid and lengthy diet required—or the motivation to do so. They obviously prefer to live with a tumor or ulcer or diabetes or whatever rather than rid themselves of it by a diet prescribed for their individual case. Remember the old saw concerning the horse and water?

Sometimes the patient, unlike the horse, knows the "life-saving water" is there, but his professional life is so arranged that he cannot (or so he believes) stick to his therapeutic diet. Many of the motion-picture stars I have treated, for instance, travel to faraway places or must attend many public functions and have meals at irregular hours; thus they find it difficult to eat properly. But when they return home, ill, exhausted, filled with tension, they immediately go on what they call "Bieler broth"—a combination of lightly cooked string beans, celery, zucchini and parsley or whatever other vegetables I've recommended for their particular ailments. Even one correct meal aids a toxin-saturated body.

The patient goes to the doctor not only for preservation of life but for as much freedom from pain and disability as it is possible to give. But when the patient will not co-operate at all, the doctor is powerless to function. When, however, a patient will co-operate, I always warn him at the beginning of the crises he will go through when he starts on his rejuvenating diet. His body undergoes a "physiological housecleaning," which was impossible while he was surfeiting himself on foods that originally created the toxemia in the fluids and tissues of his system. So he must excrete this toxic load of accumulated debris. During this preliminary fast (either of just water or of diluted vegetable broths and diluted fruit juices) he may experience more or less severe headache, nausea, vertigo, biliousness, etc., for many days. The amount of unpleasant symptoms will depend on the condition of his body. Deprived of his stimulating foods and beverages, he will experience a mild type of "withdrawal symptoms" somewhat similar to those suffered by a narcotics addict who takes the cure. The disagreeable symptoms then give way to a sense of well-being as the healing processes of the body become activated. Finally, I tell the patient that the compensation of health through judicious eating will reward him in the ratio in which he applies it.

Over the years I have found that a patient must have a sort of mission in life—something very important that he hopes to accomplish to the best of his ability—before he is really motivated to seek a cure. I can only stress the fact that *he must cure himself;* I cannot do any more than *help* the process along and try to help him adjust to his particular type of food. But the cure comes from within, and in the end it is Nature that does it. If the individual is interested enough and is really anxious to experience radiant health (possibly for the first time in his life), he co-operates. But the average person does not have any real mission in life; his off-work hours revolve about the conviviality of group eating and drinking—and as a result the undertakers are kept busy.

Unhappily, they are kept busy by too many people who should

be in the prime of life. From the start of my studies I firmly believed that principles of correct food management would, without the help of pills or nostrums, correct disease—not only cure but prevent it. But I was not then, and am not today, an evangelist beating the drums for my theories. I never limited my practice to nutrition. I delivered the babies of my patients; I took care of their children, saw them safely married and delivered their new crop of babies. General practice infuses a doctor with a feeling of devotion for his patients. He gets to know them and finds soul-satisfying rewards in caring for them.

I have never considered myself a specialist.

People came to me who were disappointed in orthodox medical treatment—especially the stimulation drugs with which they were merely whipping the tired horses imprisoned in their bodies. They came to me for dietary reform usually because they had found out as they went along that food had something to do with their disorders and symptoms. So a good many of them came *willing* to follow some dietary advice—*willing* to try to experience better health through better nutrition. Naturally that made it easier to treat them.

The average person is mightily disinclined to curtail the diet he has followed all his life. He is not aware that nearly all bad food habits are *stimulation habits:* that is, the body has almost automatically found out what makes it feel better for a half hour or so and what will mask the depression and fatigue symptoms momentarily. Some people will eat a good deal of salt, others large amounts of meat washed down with cups of strong coffee, while still others rely on sweets or a combination of foods which prove harmful in their individual cases. When I take the stimulation away, the individual feels weak and depressed and headachy temporarily while the body adjusts to the new regime and the toxic matter is eliminated. Without taking this into consideration, though, many patients decide that dietary reform just isn't for them. They came to the doctor for *immediate* relief and instead they feel worse. So they return to their stimulation habits. It is a tragic decision I cannot fight. (I will have much to say about this in later chapters.)

I hope, too, that the reader with a hazy conception of how his body works will gain understanding, at least to some degree, in this book. Every day physicians see unthinking patients who treat their bodies—the most priceless of their possessions—with the reckless abandon of a child breaking a new toy. As an article in *Life* magazine (December 7, 1962) so well puts it:

> The body . . . runs on food and oxygen much as an auto runs on gasoline and oxygen. But right there the comparison ends. If it is not to stall or splutter, the auto must be fed exactly what it needs just when it needs it. The body's fuel system, on the other hand, is subject to the whimsical tastes and cravings of its proprietor. It can handle extra food when it is already full and can go without when it is empty. And it must tolerate surprise doses of gin, smoke and red-hot chili. It does this heroic job remarkably well . . . Though people often think of the stomach as a finicky, delicate organ, it is actually so rugged it can tolerate virtually anything that is not downright poisonous or corrosive.

True, the accommodating digestive system can tolerate strange substances. But not forever. Sooner or later, depending on its present state and on hereditary health factors, it breaks down, it is invaded by disease. Its fuel-processing system as well as its transportation system through the digestive canal break down because their normal work is interfered with. When the fuel pump—or heart—is impaired, heart disease (the number-one killer in the United States) may occur. If the digestive canal is overloaded too long with improper food residues, the coronary arteries harden and a heart attack may result. If the air you breathe is polluted, you may suffer respiratory trouble. If the water you drink is too chlorinated or medicated with fluorine, your body may be irritated by the caustic action. If your teeth are neglected, you may suffer from malnutrition because you cannot eat the food you need for optimum health.

Even with an abundance of good food near at hand, most Americans rarely choose it. "The breakfast slimes, angel food cake, doughnuts and coffee, white bread and gravy cannot build an enduring nation," warned Dr. Martin H. Fischer, and a number of other medical men have echoed his words as they observed a cross section of Americans—subsisting on lifeless, overprocessed, insecticide-sprayed food; saturated with toxic matter from such stimulators as coffee, tea, alcohol, chocolate, sweetened cola drinks; medicated with stimulating pep-up drugs—men and women whose low state of health just barely keeps them alive.

Is it any wonder, then, that their bodies—do-it-yourself repair shops—have no tools with which to work?

But America's poor dietary habits aren't completely a product of the atomic age. A Frenchman, Constantin Volney, observed the diet of farmers in New England 164 years ago. And although few Frenchmen ever regard any other nation's food to be at all appetizing, it is easy to see why M. Volney termed the following menu "deplorable":

> In the morning at breakfast they douse their stomachs with a quart of hot water impregnated with tea or so slightly with coffee that it is mere colored water; and they could swallow almost without thinking hot bread half baked, toast soaked in butter, cheese of the fattest kind, slices of salt or hung beef, ham, etc., all of which is nearly insoluble. At dinner they have boiled pastes under the name of puddings, and their sauces, even for roast beef, are melted butter; then potatoes and turnips swimming in hog's lard, butter or fat. Under the name of pie or pudding, their pastry is nothing but a greasy paste, never sufficiently baked.

No wonder a flourishing industry of the day was the making of false teeth, skillfully carved from hickory wood, highly prized even today by antique collectors. But primitive man had no need of store teeth. Scientific research has shown us that he had an excellent set of teeth with which to do his own chewing.

One of man's most valuable assets throughout history has been his body's capacity to repair itself. And the same goes for animals. They possess a built-in instinct for survival. Doesn't the sick dog go outside to nibble grass on the lawn; the wounded cat lick its wounds clean; the lice-infested bird wallow in the dust? This primitive instinct, called *vis medicatrix naturae* is at the root of all the healing arts; it is as ancient as life itself, as useful to the first single-celled form of life floating in some forgotten sea a billion years ago as it is to us—the sons and daughters of that first simple living organism, today. Why, then, have we forgotten it?

3

Disease Has Many Faces

> We are the world's wealthiest country—yet one of
> the unhealthiest. We are flabby, overweight, and have
> a lot of dental caries, fluoridation notwithstanding.
> Our gastrointestinal system operates like a spluttering
> gas engine. We can't sleep; we can't get going when
> we are awake. We have neuroses; we have high blood
> pressure. Neither our hearts nor our heads last as long
> as they should. Coronary disease at the peak of life has
> hit epidemic proportions. Suicide is one of the lead-
> ing causes of death (fourth between the ages of fifteen
> and forty-four). We suffer from a plethora of the dis-
> eases of civilization.
>
> —HERBERT RATNER, M.D.

What, exactly, are these diseases of civilization? What, in fact, is
disease? Where does it come from? Why does it strike the human
body? At precisely what point does a healthy man become a sick
man? If I am to help you understand the importance of diet in your
own life, I must ask these questions and others, too.

The average individual, generally, is mystified at such queries and
has no answers, or else incorrect ones.

Isn't it strange that a person will keep in his mind such relatively
useless information as the last World Series scores, the lines of some
minor poem memorized in grammar school, the Academy Award
winners of the past five years—and be more or less ignorant of the
way his body works and why he is tormented by pain, disease and

breakdown of body organs? Does he ever think as he sees the light flashing on a firefly's tail that he is observing amazing chemical processes far more intricate than manmade experiments in an atomic laboratory?

You may pride yourself on understanding the mysteries of inertial navigation or lunar travel, but can you locate your liver? Generally not, that is, if your liver is silently going on about its amazingly complex tasks. But when it is *ailing*, you crave knowledge. As Dr. Ian Stevenson wisely observed, "If a man will not study himself when well, he must, when ill."

Ordinarily, only his body's outer surface is known to him. His intricate functional activities are felt only as a vague sense of well-being, until he is aware of that signal of distress, pain. He gets a splinter in his finger and promptly forgets it. Later, he surveys the swollen, inflamed tissues around it with annoyance. "Why does this have to happen to me today, when I'm so busy?" he asks in anger. He does not realize his body is forever fighting a biological battle for his survival; the swelling and inflammation (boil or abscess) is a wise response of the body, for they constitute a complete quarantine, a thick barricade of inflammatory tissue to prevent the enemy (microbes or poisons) from spreading further throughout the body.

Unable to use the finger, he awkwardly cuts his face while shaving. Now he is annoyed not only by the pain of his inflamed finger but by the drops of blood trickling down his face. He doesn't understand that the inflammation triggers the pain in his finger to prevent him from using it. That is a wise provision of nature—a protective device for getting the injured part out of action and ready for the body's repair materials to go to work. Casually, he accepts the drying up of the blood on his face. Does he stop to think that the blood is liquid in his body, yet at the tiny cut, it has become solid? Does this seem a miraculous thing to him—this blood-clotting mechanism which prevents all his blood from draining out? It does, to scientists studying it.

"It is highly dishonorable for a Reasonable Soul to live in so Divinely built a Mansion as the Body he resides in, altogether unacquainted with the exquisite structure of it," declared Robert Boyle (b. 1627). Unhappily, he could not have learned much scientific information about the "exquisite structure" of his "Soul's Mansion" during those early days, but the interested reader of today can, by reading any one of a number of complete guides to the machinery of the body—material which this present book, because of space limitations, can merely touch on. But, following Plato's warning, I am not suggesting that my intent is to make the patient a doctor in ten easy lessons.

To understand disease we must understand the living cell. Each of us is composed of more than a trillion cells—each one a tremendously complicated mechanism. Even today this mechanism is understood only slightly. When the body becomes diseased, its cells become abnormal in various ways. Human knowledge does not extend yet to an understanding of the operation of cells under both physiological and pathological conditions. But we do know there are two classes of disease: infectious, caused by viruses or bacteria entering the body; degenerative, caused, in general, by toxic substances manufactured by the disturbed organs themselves or by toxic material in food and air. Against both types the body strives with might and main, trying to neutralize the offending material or to free the body from factors in the environment unfavorable to it.

Probably, one supposes, the entire history of medicine began with the menace of accident, injury and disease, or *dis-ease*, as encountered by the first and highly vulnerable man in the dawn of history. The oldest evidence of illness in man is to be found in human bones, for flesh decayed, but bones survived. Examination of Egyptian mummies clearly reveals chronic rheumatism affecting joints, and spinal tuberculosis. And we have uncovered on the walls of a cave in the Pyrénées a rock painting of the Aurignacian age, some seventeen thousand years ago, of the earliest known physician —a witch doctor, wearing animal skins and a fearsome headdress made of stag's antlers.

The earliest man believed that disease was caused by demons who stole into his body (some primitive people still believe this). The ill person in primitive society was thought to be bewitched; he was ostracized and the magic powers of a medicine man or sorcerer were necessary to frighten and expel the evil spirits or demons before the victim could be restored to health.

During more civilized days in ancient Egypt, a patient taking medicine was urged to pray: "Welcome remedy! Welcome! Thou dost drive away that which is in my heart and limbs." Even in the advanced age of Plato, the belief persisted that disease was due to "the displeasure of the gods." And it was not until the human liberator Hippocrates appeared, in the Golden Age of Greece, that magic, superstition and demonology were thrown onto the waste heap. He brought the art of medicine, according to Sir William Osler, "out of the murky night of the East, heavy with phantoms, into the bright daylight of the West."

It has been said that we owe everything either to nature or to the ancient Greeks. Medically speaking, this is true. Nature, the Greeks knew, was the foremost healer. And Hippocrates taught men how to help Mother Nature in her work. He knew that disease had a cause and followed a certain course; that it could be predicted and removed from the body through certain regimens. He knew, too, that the laws of nature cannot be broken and that those laws do not change.

But the civilized learning of Hippocrates and his followers gathered dust during the Middle Ages, when superstition, magic and ignorance again held sway. The Church took over from the medicine man, the witch doctor, the tribal shaman. With the renewed belief that disease was caused by demonic possession came the treatment: prayers, exorcism, the laying on of hands, the sight of holy relics. The victim of disease recovered—or he died. But, thanks to the human body's amazing recuperative do-it-yourself powers, man frequently recovered his health despite lack of treatment or the revolting concoctions poured down his throat. One wonders how any of the disease-ridden managed to survive. That they did is a wonderful tribute to the body's many lines of defense.

The seventeenth century saw the dawn of scientific medicine, yet even by 1685 weird methods of treating the ill prevailed. Even a king, Charles II of England, was not spared. Witness this account which Drs. H. M. and A. R. Somers give in their book *Doctors, Patients and Health Insurance:*

> Once upon a time a king, while shaving, fell unconscious in his bedroom. The following treatment was employed by the royal physician. A pint of blood was extracted from his right arm; then eight ounces from the left shoulder; next an emetic, two physics, and an enema consisting of fifteen substances. Then his head was shaved and a blister raised on the scalp. To purge the brain a sneezing powder was given; then cowslip powder to strengthen it. Meanwhile more emetics, soothing drinks, and more bleeding; also a plaster of pitch and pigeon dung applied to the royal feet. Not to leave anything undone, the following substances were taken internally: melon seeds, manna, slippery elm, black cherry water, extract of lily of the valley, peony, lavender, pearls dissolved in vinegar, gentian root, nutmeg, and finally forty drops of extract of human skull. As a last resort bezoar stone was employed. But the patient died.

Patients continued to die by the thousands in the epidemics and plagues that periodically ravaged civilized nations. But when, in the latter half of the last century, Louis Pasteur and his disciples discovered that tiny organisms entered the body and caused illness, medical science was able to suppress one class of disease.

Before Pasteur, the pathologist Rudolf Virchow formulated his cellular pathology doctrine: every disease is essentially a disease of cells. According to Virchow, the body can be likened to a country of which each of its cells is a citizen. Disease, then, as Virchow saw it, is a war of the citizen cells—a war brought about by the action of enemy forces outside the body.

Other investigators hold that disease is a method of protection for the body; an adjustment to a natural phenomenon. Disease, they say, is never just a surrender to the dark forces of decay and death; it is also a fight for health. "The very concept of illness presupposes a clash between forces of aggression and our defenses," observed Dr. Hans Selye in *The Stress of Life.* Pain, though an unwelcome intruder, serves a useful purpose. In disease, it is a warning given by nature to enforce rest as an aid to healing. It is also a warning that we may have suffered an injury. The nerve endings, receptors, transmit a message along the nerve pathways by electrical impulses to the brain, and we experience pain as a reaction. A variety of sensory stimuli can trigger pain: chemical; mechanical, such as twisting of a limb or pressure; thermal, as extreme cold or heat; or electrical. When there is inflammation because of disease or injury, there is usually a combination of mechanical pressure and chemical irritation. Pain is always a warning that something is amiss; thus, to the physician, it is one of the most important symptoms of disease.

The phone rings at night and you stub your toe in the dark. The sharp sensation makes you wonder why man must be afflicted with pain. And your wonder turns to despair as you observe cancer causing a loved one to suffer. Yet pain, from a mere twinge to the most exquisite torture of a kidney stone, is the body's best protective device. For example, it makes you keep a broken arm quiet so that your do-it-yourself repair shop of a body can get to work.

The stricken body always seeks to return to a state of health— to be free of the nagging pains, stabbing sensations, feelings of pressure, vague aches, intestinal disturbances which many people accept as a normal way of life.

I do not agree that this is normal.

To me, true health is much more. It is achieved by following the laws of nature; when you break them, illness results. Health is not something bestowed on you by beneficent nature at birth; it is achieved and maintained only by active participation in well-defined rules of healthful living—rules which you may be disregarding every day.

Physicians abroad comment on the fact that Americans take more medicines and submit to more surgery and inoculations than do natives of any other country. Even so, Americans are more filled with anxiety about the state of their health than any other people. In the materialistic civilization in this country, we tend to think of health as something that comes in a capsule purchased over the counter in a drugstore, instead of as a state which we attain by following the laws of nature. We believe that anyone who can afford it can be healthy.

They rarely see it, but physicians know what the old-fashioned term "glowing health" really means. They do not, however, agree on the causes of disease. For generations doctors have been debating this subject; like soldiers, they are drawn up in opposing camps, vehemently arguing that disease is caused by X or Y or Z.

4

Cornerstones in My House
of Health

> Only by understanding the wisdom of the body shall
> we attain that mastery of disease and pain which shall
> enable us to relieve the burden of mankind.
>
> —WILLIAM HARVEY, M.D.

In the last chapter I left a large group of puzzled medical men obstinately debating the question: What causes disease?

I, too, have my theories on disease and my remedies.

But please do not misunderstand; these are not merely *my own theories* and *my own remedies*—they are culled from the centuries, the cream skimmed off the milk of time. Although part of the healing art for generations, they have been unaccountably neglected in our present miracle-drug-ridden day. If I have done one thing, it is to gather them together, dust them off and then determine if they will work today. They do work. Magnificently.

Nature made man a generally perfect machine. But man, through ignorance, fear and greed has thrown a monkey wrench into that machine. Health is simple; few have it. Why?

Because we do not give nature an opportunity to reveal her story. I hope to make you aware of these secrets of nature as you become convinced that *food, not drugs, is your best medicine.*

In this book you will discover which are the harmful and which the helpful foods and how the body reacts to both in health and in illness. And this is of overwhelming importance. It is my hope that through an understanding of body chemistry and food therapy you will become as convinced as I am that (1) disease is based on an improper diet and (2) that a proper diet can best restore the ill person to health without the necessity of employing drugs or questionable surgery.

Let me give you a few quick examples. Zucchini, a member of the squash family, is a bland vegetable, especially rich in sodium. And since sodium, of all the alkaline elements of the body, is the most important, it follows that zucchini is a most healthful vegetable. The liver is the storehouse of sodium, an element necessary to maintain the acid-base equilibrium of the body. Without this acid-base balance, good health is impossible to maintain. The simple, bland zucchini, used as both food and medicine, is an ideal way to restore a sodium-exhausted liver.

As valuable in the diet as zucchini may be, it is not a cure-all. Even a bland broth made from it or from string beans, for example, would be too corrosive, irritating and alkaline for the sensitive, denuded membrane in the bowel of a bleeding-gastric-ulcer patient. For him I prescribe tiny cakes of ordinary yeast, not as a medicine, but simply as another vegetable in his diet. Where vegetable broths of the best kind would still be too caustic to blanket a bleeding ulcer, yeast diluted in a little milk or water is excellent, rich in vegetable vitamins, soft in the intestines and correct in alkalinity. I have given as many as twenty-two cakes a day to bleeding-ulcer patients, and in three or four days the ulcer has ceased to bleed and is healed.

You will discover many such body-restoring foods listed in these pages—foods to use therapeutically—for my aim is to make you well if you are ill or to show you how to continue in health, simply and inexpensively. But I must warn you that you will not find here any "magic foods" which supposedly keep the mountain peasants in some obscure Asian village in miraculous health. I leave that to the health faddists, the vitamin- and food-supplement peddlers, the medical sideshow drummers who seek to exploit the ever present desire of sick people for a panacea.

My method of treatment, the product of long neglected medical truths combined with the most up-to-date laboratory techniques, is based on health instead of disease. Whereas other medical men appear to accept sickness, physical decrepitude and degenerative disease as a natural circumstance following middle age, I consider them a consequence of unnatural living habits; improper high-caloric diets; stimulating drugs. And I have never wanted to tell a patient "how to live with" arthritis or asthma or ulcers or migraine but how to rid himself of his disability forever. During a half century of practice I have labored to one end: to free people from disease and to keep them out of my office. Yet the sick, discouraged after endless pills and potions, shots and surgery, come to me in a seemingly endless stream. And when they learn to co-operate with and not fight Nature, I bid them a fond farewell.

If I were to ask you, "Which men do you consider history's greatest benefactors?" your list no doubt would include the French chemist Louis Pasteur, the first to declare that disease is caused by germs, tiny organisms, carried from person to person. But what if I were to tell you that I disagree with Pasteur's germ theory? To say anything against the venerable Louis Pasteur—"the most perfect man who ever entered the kingdom of science"—is to most people as socially unacceptable as maligning motherhood. Nevertheless, my own research (and much research done before my time) has shown that the germ theory of disease does not tell the whole story, and that pasteurization of milk destroys much of its nutritional value. Since you have undoubtedly been taught as children that germs alone cause disease, it is not easy to divorce yourself from this philosophy. Undoubtedly, too, you have been warned against drinking unpasteurized milk.

But as far back as 1883 John Shaw Billings, the American authority on public health, was saying: "It is important to remember ... that the mere introduction of germs into the living organism does not ensure their multiplication, or the production of disease. The condition of the organism itself has much influence on the result . . . Pasteur has certainly made a hasty generalization in declaring that the only condition which determines an epidemic is the greater or less abundance of germs."

Despite proof to the contrary, many doctors still cling to the germ theory of disease and to the necessity of drugs to combat germs. They point out that smallpox, diphtheria, typhoid fever and pneumonia have been conquered. That is true; no one can quarrel with them on that score. But such major chronic disorders as cancer, heart disease, diabetes, arteriosclerosis, nephrosis and hepatitis have increased eightfold. Scientific medicine, while suppressing deadly infectious diseases by the use of modern drugs, antibiotics and immunizations, has not been able to reduce the killing power of another equally frightening set of diseases.

Instead of blindly following Pasteur (as so many medical men have done) I asked myself: Is invasion of the tissues from without —by bacteria and viruses—the *only* way by which human tissues are injured? Can disease come from other means? Shouldn't man's constitutional and environmental conditions also be considered? Hasn't the time come to expand our notions of illness and treatment beyond Pasteur's bacterial infection theory? Can it be possible that germs are merely a *concomitant of disease*, present in all of us but able to multiply in a sick individual because of disturbed function?

In seeking answers to these questions, I left Pasteur and his tiny organisms and went off on another road. And I found I was not a lonely traveler. I shall not take the time now to detail my own painstaking research into body chemistry, but will merely say that I came to the conclusion that germs do not *initiate* a diseased state of the body but appear later after a person becomes ill. In my experimental and laboratory work I found myself irresistibly drawn back to Hippocrates, who believed that disease was the result of some mismanagement of the environment. Since the chief environment was chemical and centered around the food consumed by the individual, it was only natural that when disease occurred, the finger of suspicion pointed to the fact that there had been some improper, unnatural food in the diet.

As I said in the Preface, medicine today is in a dark age. And one area of darkness is the ignorance and apathy shown by many of my colleagues in the field of dietetics. In this regard Hippocrates was an enlightened physician. His first step in maintaining health was *regimen*, or a regulated mode of life. He knew that nature made the cure and that the doctor's role was to assist nature. He believed that the diseased body needed a period of rest—not only physical rest, but chemical rest, which he considered even more important. Chemical rest could be achieved only by withholding food, thus giving the organs of the body an opportunity to discharge accumulated waste products and thereby cleanse themselves.

Thomas Sydenham called the "English Hippocrates," after a lifetime of practice, put this whole concept of disease into one simple sentence: "*Disease*," he declared, "*is nothing else but an attempt on the part of the body to rid itself of morbific matter*" [italics added].

Sydenham lived in the seventeenth century. Yet these words are as true today as they were then. The Dutch clinician Hermann Boerhaave, following in Sydenham's footsteps, declared: "Disease is cured with the help of Nature, [by] neutralization and excretion of morbific matter." Just prior to Pasteur's day Rudolf Virchow, in his pioneer work on cellular pathology, maintained that the health of body cells depended on their chemical make-up and this chemical make-up depended in turn upon the kind of food eaten by the individual. "If I could live my life over again," stated Virchow, "I would devote it to proving that germs seek their natural habitat—diseased tissue—rather than being the cause of diseased tissue; e.g. mosquitoes seek the stagnant water, but do not *cause* the pool to become stagnant." Unfortunately, Virchow's theory struck an unsympathetic note, since man has never taken kindly to having his eating habits changed or reformed. While the mechanisms of digestion and absorption are inherited mechanisms, the eating habits of an individual are learned habits. Understandably, they are difficult to break.

And when Pasteur came along, with his spectacular demonstrations of the germ theory, the public, as well as the doctors, cast out the teachings of Virchow with relief. Here, they exclaimed loudly, were the real demons! Did it matter that man remained a creature of bad living habits? No, for now he could remain so with a clear conscience, because fighting germs gave him something exciting to do.

My system of treatment is far from exciting; it is the application of common sense and modern scientific research. But most Americans are actionists; when ill, they enjoy doing something, like gulping pills, or having something done to them, like undergoing surgery. Told to rest, to abstain from irritating food and drugs, to allow the body to heal itself, they become skeptical and fearful; then they seek a doctor who will *do* something. So modern medicine, for the most part, has cast aside Hippocrates' simple and undramatic method of treating illness by *regimen*—proper food, rest and fresh air. But a few still heed his words, spoken twenty-four centuries ago when the great physician-teacher told his medical students on the sea-swept island of Cos that disease is not only *pathos* (suffering) but *ponos* (toil), or the urgency of the body to regain its normal, healthy state. This is called *vis medicatrix naturae* —the healing power of nature which cures from within. If more serious measures than regimen were called for, Hippocrates had a second line of defense: medicines; a third, if deemed necessary, was surgery. Today, mostly at the insistence of patients, American doctors have reversed Hippocrates' procedure, and the surgeon is the star of the medical show. (Let me hasten to add that I am not against surgery when it is absolutely necessary.)

The theory that his illness is the result of toxemia *inside* his body is not a pleasant one for the patient; Pasteur's theory that disease is caused by organisms from *outside* the body is easier to accept. For then he can pity himself as merely a victim of a ruthless enemy and cry: "Why did this have to happen to me?"

Over and over I explain to patients, "Your pain, misery and illness result from your own dietary mistakes and drugs. You are suffering because you are filled with toxic wastes caused by your diet of poorly selected food filled with artificial flavorings, preservatives, synthetics, over-processed ingredients—too much stimulating food, too few natural vitamins from vegetables and fruits. Even if you selected wholesome, natural foods, they were probably improperly prepared, boiled to death or overheated in oil, then covered with harmful condiments. The normal chemistry of your digestion is upset not only by these toxic wastes but also by harmful drugs, unhealthy living habits that include lack of exercise. So, highly poisonous materials—toxins—which have stagnated in your blood, impair the filters and eliminative organs, chief of which are the kidneys, liver, bowels and skin."

These toxins are the villains—the real cause of disease; they must be eliminated if the body is to be restored to health.

Illness, then, as we know it, is nothing more or less than a terrific "attempt on the part of the body to rid itself of morbific [toxic] matter" [italics added].

This is the first cornerstone on which I build my house of health.

The body's "terrific attempt" to burn up these waste products results in fever. And it is the changes (usually destructive) in the organs being used as avenues of emergency vicarious elimination which constitute the pathology, or conditions and processes of a disease.

Since "emergency vicarious elimination" is probably new to you, let me explain it, for it is another important cornerstone of my treatment in the fight against disease; I will have much to say of it in future chapters.

The liver and the kidneys are important eliminative organs. For the liver, the natural avenue of elimination, of course, is through the bowel; for the kidneys, through the bladder and urethra.

However, when the liver is congested and cannot perform its eliminative function, waste matter (toxins) is thrown into the blood stream. Similarly, when the kidneys are inflamed, toxins are also dammed up in the blood. Toxic blood must discharge its toxins or the person dies, so nature uses vicarious avenues of elimination or substitutes. The lungs, therefore, will take over the task of eliminating some of the wastes that should have gone through the kidneys, or the skin will take over for the liver. It stands to reason that the lungs do not make very good kidneys. From the irritation caused by the elimination of poison through this "vicarious" channel, we can get bronchitis, pneumonia or tuberculosis, as is determined by the particular *chemistry* of the poison being eliminated. Thus we can say that the lungs are acting *vicariously* for the kidneys or are being called into play, under duress, as substitute kidneys. In the same way, if the bile poisons in the blood come out through the skin, we get the various irritations of the skin, resulting in the many skin diseases, or through the mucous membranes (inside skin) as the various catarrhs, or through the skin as boils, carbuncles, acne, etc. Thus, the skin is substituting for the liver, or a vicarious elimination is occurring through the skin.

Following this line of thinking, the name of a disease is based upon a description, macro- and microscopic, of the changes in the organs being used as emergency avenues of elimination. After the cells have been damaged by toxic wastes, it is easy for bacteria, as scavengers, to attack and devour the weakened, injured and dead cells.

Disease, then, as I see it is an unnatural elimination process. In order to speed along or facilitate the natural elimination process of the toxic material and return the patient to health, I found necessary either (1) complete abstention from food (fasting for a few days or longer) or (2) abstention from those foods which created the patient's toxemia.

In seeking methods of eliminating toxemia from the system, I turned my attention to the endocrine, or ductless, glands of the body. Specifically for my interests, though there are others, the liver, thyroid, adrenal and pituitary glands became the object of my research. A long period of study (both here and in Europe), along original lines, of the endocrine glands, particularly of the functions of the liver, brought to light just how I could use the endocrine system to aid in eliminating the toxemia poisoning the system of the patient. (The endocrine glands, once a fashionable subject for medical attention, have been unaccountably neglected of late. Physicians at one time, for instance, passed out dessicated thyroid tablets in all sorts of dosages to their overweight patients; when it proved useless in weight reduction, they lost interest in all the endocrine glands.)

This study of the endocrine system led me to another and very important area of research: the stimulating effects on the human system of various foods and such inorganic non-food substances as salt, etc. This stimulating effect of certain foods is directly related to the endocrine glands. I will have much to say about this later on, but let me ask you a question: How many of you can't start your day without steaming cups of strong coffee, which is in no sense a food? How many of you are relying more and more on the "coffee break" to get you through the morning? No doubt, you "enjoy" it for its stimulating value. When you are young and active, you eliminate the toxic coffee acids through the urine. But later, as the kidneys gradually deteriorate with age, those acids pile up in your system drop by drop. You feel fatigued, headachy, depressed, so you drink more coffee to get through the day. Momentarily you feel better, able to fight the world, because you are *whipping* your endocrine glands (usually the adrenal glands) to produce this false sense of exhilaration. Your sense of well-being is a mask hiding the truth. How long can you continue whipping the endocrine glands? Only until their inevitable breakdown.

Because I have seen so many stimulation-whipped endocrine systems, I studied them exhaustively, beginning with my own, harmed not by coffee but by salt. To most of my patients my theories relating to stimulation and to the whole subject of toxins in the body were so revolutionary that they necessitated detailed explanation before they could be accepted. And I hope that as we share these explanations, you too will accept them.

Toxemia is caused by improper foods. The organs then are forced to become emergency streams of vicarious elimination to discharge these toxic wastes. The endocrine glands are called into action to aid in eliminating toxic poisons from the system. To gain an understanding of disease from this viewpoint we must consider the food eaten, the liver, kidneys and endocrine glands of the man eating it and the social environment in which he lives.

Food eaten today is about as far removed from the natural diet of man as man is from his primitive jungle. Man, however, still has approximately the same digestive apparatus and liver as his remote ancestors. If he lives on natural food, his liver remains efficient; if he fills his stomach with hot breads, hot dogs, chili, doughnuts washed down with strong coffee, his outraged liver cannot do its work. Whether his liver breaks down early or late depends upon how good an organ it was at birth. But break down it will, and when it fails to filter and neutralize toxins from the blood, an extra line of defense must come into play. This defense is carried on by the endocrine glands, which try to direct these toxins into other eliminative organs. The principal endocrine glands called upon for this effort are the pituitary, which lies at the base of the brain, the thyroid, situated in the neck, and the adrenals, which fit like a cap over each kidney.

Glands of internal secretion then are pressed into hyperfunction, forced to manufacture more of their secretion. However, since the amount of a gland's secretion is in exact ratio to the volume of blood entering it, the gland is enlarged by this extra blood supply, which often can have disastrous physical consequences.

The pituitary gland, for example, does not have much room in which to swell, encased as it is in a bony cup at the base of the skull. If this receptacle is congenitally small or deformed by rickets in early life, very little swelling can take place without creating a pressure on the gland within its box. This pressure can cause alarming symptoms. Four different diseased states, all arising from a toxemia of the blood, can result from the pressure: migraine headache, the common type of epilepsy, acromegaly (tremendous overgrowth or gigantism) and blindness.

There are many cases in my files of migraine and epilepsy—cases in which the distressing symptoms have been arrested and the body restored to health. This was accomplished by taking the excessive dietary burden off the liver, which then was able to cleanse the blood stream and restore a balance between the pituitary, thyroid and adrenal glands.

The medical history of most of my patients afflicted with migraine shows that they have suffered the searing pain of periodic migraine headaches since childhood. They come to me in their thirties and forties and fifties. I have found that where no drugs are involved, the migraine, in practically all cases, is really an *alcoholic* type of headache. This will, no doubt, startle migraine sufferers. But, let me hasten to add, the alcohol does not come from too many martinis before dinner; it is manufactured in the patient's own stomach. It results from the fermentation of the sugars and starches in that patient's diet. This alcohol is more harmful than bottled spirits. The whiskey drinker doesn't have to swallow fusel oil and all the other organic alcohols formed in the process; he just drinks ethyl alcohol. But alcohol made in the intestines has among its ingredients sour mash and other products very toxic to the body.

In treating patients suffering from migraine I have found that when I delete sugars and starches and increase certain natural antidotes in the diet which help eliminate the surplus of poisons, they *seldom have another headache.* Their gratitude is but one of the many joys a physician discovers in the practice of medicine.

I have seen acromegaly, or gigantism, arrested by erasing the underlying toxemia; but this is effective only during adolescence. Pressure blindness, too, can result from excessive swelling of the pituitary gland caused by food toxemia or by a toxic drug. In many cases penicillin overstimulates the pituitary gland and results in impaired vision.

Just as hypersecretion of pituitary hormones can manifest itself in illness, so can hypersecretion of the thyroid gland. This gland, located at the base of the neck, controls all functions of the body's three layers of skin: the outer skin, called the hide; the inner skin, called the mucous membrane; and a middle skin, the serous membrane, which lines the pleural, pericardial, peritoneal and cranial cavities and also those of the joints.

The normal function of the outer skin is to exhale gases, sweat out water and certain toxic salty substances and oil itself and its hair with special oil glands. The vicarious elimination, which results from forcefully exuding gases, acid sweat, and toxic oils and greases through the outer skin, has supplied names to enough diseases to fill a large dermatology textbook. Chronic eczema, ichthyosis and psoriasis are common examples. Skin diseases, which are really signs of toxic irritation, respond well to a treatment, dietary and local, directed toward neutralization and elimination of the offending poisons. This brings the hyperthyroidism under control.

The inner skin, or mucous membrane, normally secretes a clear mucus which keeps the membranes moist and, with the aid of the flagellated lining cells, propels irritants and foreign bodies toward a point where they can be eliminated. Under duress, the thyroid gland may force toxins out through the mucous cells.

When only the superficial cells of the inner skin are involved and the secretion is watery, we have a disease characterized by a serous exudation called a cold or catarrh. As the deeper layers are affected, the discharge becomes muco-purulent (mucus and pus), purulent (pure pus) or purulent-hemorrhagic (blood and pus). Under these headings would come such diseases as sinusitis, bronchitis, gastritis, enteritis, appendicitis, tonsillitis, mastitis, cervicitis, pyelitis and any other "ites" where inflammation of the mucous or serous membrane occurs.

Vicarious elimination through the middle skin results in such diseases as arthritis, neuritis, peritonitis, pericarditis, encephalitis, meningitis, bursitis and iritis. *These diseases are all inflammations and are due to a forced elimination of toxins.* I have found that the only method of curing or alleviating them is to neutralize the toxins by diet in order to relieve the congested and disturbed liver by rest (rest, that is, from improper food) and to facilitate elimination of poisons through the *natural* channels chosen by nature for that kind of work, such as the kidneys, liver, lungs, skin and bowels.

The adrenal glands were long regarded as emergency glands. It was believed earlier that they poured out their internal secretion only when man, confronted by a dangerous situation, had to resort to "fight or flight." Later, it was shown that this secretion is so vitally necessary that man cannot live for four seconds if it has left his blood. Witness the sudden death from cyanide poisoning, which puts a stop to all oxidation in the body. The adrenal secretion is the agent that makes oxidation possible.

Oxidation is the fire of life. So important is this adrenal secretion, therefore, that the body has extra depots for manufacture and storage, such as the brain and the great nerve ganglia, the posterior pituitary, the sex glands and scattered areas throughout the kidneys. This explains why some animals, and occasionally men, are able to live after extirpation of the adrenals.

The chemical process of filtration of toxins through the kidneys depends upon oxidation, which is literally a process of burning. The close proximity of the adrenals to the kidneys and the great nerve ganglia of the solar plexus suggests that one of the most vital functions of the kidneys depends upon oxidation. Here again, under duress, the kidney can be forced by the adrenals into the function of vicarious elimination, even to the point of destroying itself and elevating the blood pressure until a heart attack or other circulatory damage results.

Another adrenal function is to regulate the strength of muscle tone. This includes the bowel muscle as well as the skeletal muscles. With good bowel muscle tone, bowel function is perfect, effortless and regular. Adrenal types, that is, individuals who are dominated by their adrenal glands, seldom suffer from constipation as long as the chemistry of the liver remains normal. When an adrenal type becomes toxic from indigestion, elimination may be rapid and complete through bowel movements or even diarrhea. It is my belief, therefore, that the diseases resulting from adrenal hyperactivity are the diarrheas, the various forms of kidney trouble, cancer and many others, including a monstrous type of obesity. These states, unless the tissues are irreparably damaged, respond to the same type of treatment described for pituitary and thyroid disorders.

Although my medical theories are based mainly on my own observations and conclusions which have stood the test of time, I have not hesitated to use the most up-to-date scientific advances in today's medicine. In my intense desire to bring new hope of relief to my patients, I have availed myself of the giant strides in the sciences of chemistry and bacteriology to help clear up some of the perplexing problems of how toxic wastes affect the system. As I stated, I have spent much time in the laboratory probing deeply into the science of endocrinology to learn if it could suggest certain paths through which toxemia in the body could be eliminated.

Utilizing the old as well as the new is not, to me, a paradoxical situation, for I believe we have much to learn from long forgotten historical medical experience as well as from today's scientific inquiry.

Though the cornerstone of my treatment goes back to Hippocrates, from two great physicians of the seventeenth century—Sydenham and Boerhaave—I learned much. I found other leaders, both European and American, who, in spite of neglect and even outright denunciation by entrenched medical opinion, still raised their voices in behalf of the theory of toxemia at a time when the hold of Pasteurian dogma was strong. Before World War I, such a man was Dr. J. H. Tilden, founder of a health institution in Denver and author of *Toxemia Explained*. His working tools were fasting, cleansing diets and rational living. In his day biochemistry was in its infancy, therefore his greatest proof rested upon empirical experience. Although his practice was nation-wide, throughout his career he battled mightily against orthodoxy, "the iron yoke of conformity," as William Osler expressed it. Later, Dr. George S. Weger, a Johns Hopkins graduate and pupil of Tilden, took up the torch in behalf of the role of toxemia in disease. He was the author of *The Genesis and Control of Disease* and headed a very successful health school in Redlands, California. It was with a profound sense of gratitude that I recently shared in an honor accorded these two fine men when my name was added to a Chair of Nutrition named for them—The Tilden-Weger-Bieler Chair of Dietetic Medicine at Columbia University's Goldwater Memorial Hospital.

It was my privilege to add a few bricks to the basic foundations laid down by these pioneers—to use the newer findings of chemistry and endocrinology in clearing up many previously unexplainable problems. I shall mention only one in passing, the present enigma of the relationship of cholesterol to arterial disease. Very early I was aware of the cholesterol problem—long before it became a household word. (A later chapter will discuss this in detail.) Through original research I determined what foods supply the chemical ingredients that can be built up into cholesterol; I also

determined what is one of the most important functions of cholesterol. Most valuable of all, I have discovered which foods build a
chemically pure, natural cholesterol and which foods result in an
unnatural, pathological type—a type which does not wear well in
the body tissues since it causes much arterial damage. Like a structure built with improperly mixed concrete, the blood vessels crumble
or are eroded when they are deprived of natural cholesterol.

Orthodox medicine follows well-defined paths; I have explored
little-traveled roads and byways, especially in the field of body
chemistry. And although some of my conclusions have been received with skepticism and even hostility by conservative physicians, I have never flinched under attack. For I have living proof
of my theories—patients who came to me ill and discouraged and
left restored in body and spirits. I admit mine is not an easy or
pleasant cure, as is popping pills into your mouth. Complete bed
rest, while fasting on diluted fruit juices and vegetable broths, isn't
particularly appealing even for a few days. And living thereafter
on a diet restricted in starches or proteins or fats or salt (as the case
may be) is even less appealing as a way of life. But isn't it better
than dragging through years of self-inflicted subnormal health, a
victim of migraine or digestive complaints or asthma, etc.?

I do not mind being labeled "controversial" or worse, for much
of the material in this book is original and does not conform to current patterns of medical thought. Throughout medical history many
advances in healing have been achieved in the face of intense opposition by those with closed minds. Walter Bagehot tells us that
"the pain of a new idea is one of the greatest pains in human nature
. . . after all, your favorite notions may be wrong, your firmest be-
liefs ill-founded."

There is, however, a small but growing band of physicians who
are willing to accept a "new idea." In medical school they were
taught to consider sickness only in terms of germs—now they are
revising their thinking as they discover unmistakable evidence that
malfunctions of the body itself lead to diseased states. In following less conventional and more independent lines of inqufry, they
have left the germ theory of disease far behind. True, they find

this new path an unpopular and rather lonely one. Yet it is one my own research and experience over many years has forced me to follow.

Let me add a word of caution: since what you find here will be new and revolutionary, and since, in all likelihood, your doctors have prescribed drugs but never discussed toxemia with you, you may find yourself a bit skeptical in accepting my premise that the wrong foods cause disease and the right foods cure disease. But let me assure you that after you free yourself of your "drug" hypnosis, you are taking a major step up the ladder of well-being. It is true that many drugs pep you up at first, but soon the added stimulation only further depletes the exhausted body.

Medical literature is filled with conflicting ideas on what causes disease—each with its fervent supporters. Those on the other side of the fence from me hold that food has little to do with preparing the pathway for disease. They believe that the body can utilize anything to good account except poisons. So they condemn the theories of toxemia, intestinal putrefaction, auto-intoxication as "faddist" and remain unwilling to take them seriously.

"In general," declared Dr. Logan Clendening in *The Human Body*, "what you want to eat will be good for you. 'What one relishes, nourishes,' was a maxim of Poor Richard. Instinct is a wise physician. The appetite is a wonderfully sensitive instrument, a safe compass. It keeps most of us exactly where we ought to be in weight and strength."

This, in view of statistics showing that the average American is overweight! Is his appetite a sensitive instrument when he is surrounded by the greatest food supply in the world? The average American, generally, has no conception of what it means to enjoy normal good health. How could he? He has never known it. Just as there are levels of disease, so are there levels of health.

As Louis Herber, in *Our Synthetic Environment*, warns:

We are exchanging health for mere survival. We have begun to measure man's biological achievements, not in terms of his ability to lead a vigorous, physically untroubled life, but in terms of his ability to preserve his mere existence in an increasingly distorted environment. Today, survival often entails ill health and rapid physical degeneration. We are prepared to accept the fact that a relatively young individual will suffer from frequent headaches and digestive disturbances, continual nervous tension, insomnia, a persistent "cigarette cough," a mouthful of decaying teeth, and respiratory ailments every winter. We expect his physique to acquire the rotundity of a barrel shortly after the onset of middle age; we find nothing extraordinary in the fact that he is incapable of running more than a few yards without suffering loss of breath or walking a few miles without suffering exhaustion.

According to the findings of the United States Commission on Chronic Illness (published by Harvard University, 1957): "In 1950 an estimated 28 million Americans were suffering from ... chronic disease. There is no reason to think that this number has decreased." Other statistics point to the possibility that since 1950 the actual number of persons suffering from chronic diseases has increased far faster than the population. Medical science is acutely aware of this shocking figure. I chose to believe, after many years of patient research, that when the strain of faulty living habits, reliance on stimulating drugs, incorrect diet and poor environment have broken down the filters of the body, a toxemia naturally develops which results in what is commonly known as disease. The basic cause of disease, therefore, is the toxemia. The name of the disease describes the damage done by the toxemia. This belief goes back to ancient days, and it is opposed to the attempt to overcome disease by either powerful and dangerous drugs or risky surgery. The treatment of toxemia, such as I have discussed with you in these pages, is extremely simple: it is not dramatic; it does not cure overnight. But *cure* it will if the patient co-operates with both nature and with his physician.

Today, the science of medicine is directing itself to a more detailed chemical examination of disease based upon a foundation more rational than that of demons, fear or even germs. Today, gradually, we are returning to the poet Milton's wise words: "Accuse not Nature; she hath done her part; do thou but thine."

And now let us examine by what means our incomparable human body does its part against the onslaught of disease.

5

Digestion: First Line of Defense Against Disease

Things sweet to taste prove in digestion sour.
—SHAKESPEARE, KING RICHARD II

The round and butterballish man in the Los Angeles cafeteria methodically loads his tray: cream of corn soup, two white rolls and four pats of butter, a dish of spaghetti flanked by meatballs. His eyes hesitate momentarily over the crisp green salads, but he resolutely marches on to select apple pie with ice cream, coffee with sugar and cream. Behind him, the lanky greyhound man selects a bowl of vegetable soup, broiled lamb chops, string beans, a large mixed green salad without dressing, a glass of skimmed milk and baked apple.

As one judges from the above: man is both carnivorous (meat eating) and herbivorous (plant eating); he is also omnivorous (everything eating!). His body, a chemical engine, accepts all the food it is fed. Some it discards violently by vomiting or diarrhea; some, from the large economy-size package fed it, it stores in fat reservoirs, a cushion against leaner times; some it gratefully uses to fire its countless tiny cell furnaces, after painstaking and marvelously complex biochemical treatment. If the energy output in the food most recently fed it is not high enough, the body insistently calls for more, and a raid on the refrigerator probably follows. If the body calls insistently for food and its owner, lost on a stormy mountain top, feeds it only melted snow, the starving body uncomplainingly uses up the fat deposits and then its own tissues for fuel. After every bit which can be spared is utilized, the engine sputters, runs down and death ensues. Disease and breakdown also result if the internal-combustion engine is stoked with the wrong kind of fuel too many times.

The digestive system is really a chemical refinery which manufactures its own fuels and delivers energy from the raw materials provided it: proteins, fats, carbohydrates (broken down into starches and sugars), vitamins and minerals. The whole process of digestion takes place in the alimentary canal. In an adult, it comprises approximately a thirty-foot-long hollow tube which begins at the mouth where food is chewed and acted upon by the saliva and ends at the anus where certain wastes are eliminated from the body. Along this continuous tube, which can be likened to an assembly line or conveyor belt, are stations where the microscopic chemists convert foodstuffs for the body's use by breaking down, diluting and dissolving as well as by adding some chemicals and removing others.

Some of the food Americans eat is natural and useful; other elements are useless or downright harmful. In many cases the rugged, resilient digestive system must cope not only with the stressful conditions of modern life but with a staggering amount and variety of food, beverages, alcohol, caffeine and nicotine as well as a flood of patent medicines, pills and powders designed for real or imaginary digestive malfunctions or constipation.

In the mouth the food particles meet their first digestive enzymes —highly specialized protein molecules which act as catalysts in aiding body processes or speeding them along. (Metabolism, the sum of the processes by which the body's fuel is converted to energy, relies heavily on enzymes, one of the basic keys of life. If their orderly reactions are interfered with, the cellular engines misfire and illness results.) The stomach secretions, the enzymes from the pancreas, the liver and the glands lining the small intestine all act on the passing food particles.

All of the food that has been subjected to the action of the enzymes and ferments and other catalytic agents of reduction in the mouth and stomach is now spread out, as it were, upon a huge carpet, many yards square. This area is the actual lining of the small intestine, which is about twenty-six feet long and covered with millions of frond-shaped villi, like little fingers in constant motion swinging back and forth, protruding from the mucosa or lining of the small intestine. Even as the grooves of a long-playing phonograph record are often more than a mile in length, so the millions of villi enlarge the absorbing surface of the small intestine. Natural sugar, in the form of glucose, as well as unnatural sugar, natural and unnatural minerals, fatty and amino acids (proteins), are spread upon this "carpet."

When the chemistry is abnormal because of the ingestion of food that ferments or putrefies in the small intestine, the resulting products are irritating to the delicate lining of the bowel. The bowel either tries to get rid of the irritations quickly, which results in a diarrhea, or puts a spastic clamp on the intestines to keep them from proceeding further, resulting in stasis or constipation.

Thus the small intestine, with its rich lining of extremely delicate and sensitive cells, can be classified as *the body's first line of defense*—fighting against the absorption of unnatural and detrimental food elements. Repeated absorption of these harmful elements produces in time an inflammation and a destruction of much of the tender lining. It is precisely then that the blood in the villi becomes so overcharged with toxic elements that these harmful materials enter the blood stream.

As the digested food particles are spread upon the intestinal carpet of villi for absorption, two very important problems present themselves: the *quantity* of the food material and the *quality*.

When too much food is eaten—such as selected by the butterball man at the opening of this chapter—it follows that too much is absorbed (rich, fatty, difficult-to-digest food makes up 40 percent of the average American diet), for villi have no regulating mechanism to indicate how much to absorb. The result is that the individual becomes either obese or ill. The illness can be acute or chronic, depending upon the glands of internal secretion. As far back as ancient Rome the dangers of overeating were recognized. The Romans were gourmets who realized that it was necessary to disgorge a great part of what they enjoyed at their exotic banquets if they wished to retain good health—or even to continue their epicurean way of life. And so they employed female attendants with receptacles for catching the vomit on these occasions. Perhaps they took seriously Hippocrates' aphorism that the very obese die earlier than the very slender.

Now, as to the *quality* of food, it has long been observed that the "mono-diet," or eating of one kind of food at a time, greatly eases digestion, especially for weak or sick people. Although today the mixing of various foods in a meal is the subject of controversy in the medical profession, throughout history the mono-diet was practiced with good results. Hippocrates prescribed milk alone for those suffering from tuberculosis. Many modern doctors follow the theories of such pioneers as Dr. J. H. Salisbury, who recommended meat alone for the relief of many diseases. Dr. William Beaumont, the young Army surgeon who in 1822 began his celebrated experiments on gastric digestion, used as his subject a fur trapper named Alexis St. Martin, whose stomach wall had been shot away. Through the hole in his patient's stomach, Beaumont observed the gastric distress which followed what is today called a "well-balanced meal." His book, though hard to find, is still one of the masterpieces of digestive study.

Well balanced or poorly chosen, foodstuff enters the alimentary canal three or more times a day. The villi, unless they are too inflamed, cannot help absorbing the food particles as they come along. Proteins, carbohydrates, fats and minerals enter the blood and lymph. Many millions of words have been written about the proteins and their amino acids, called the building blocks of the body. They are more fully discussed in later chapters.

I believe that cells, called small lymphocytes, carry the food necessary for the growth and reproduction of body cells. This food is protein in nature, but before it can be utilized by the body cells an iodine value must be imparted to it by the thyroid gland. This happens in a most fascinating way and can be followed by tracing one of these lymphocytes as it courses through the body.

Each one of the villi contains two sets of vessels: blood vessels and lymph vessels. The lymph vessels are the right-of-way for the lymphocytes and other white blood cells. They seldom contain red blood cells, although white corpuscles are normally found in small numbers in the blood contained in the blood vessels.

During digestion great numbers of lymphocytes enter the lymph vessels. In order to have an available supply of these cells nature has placed the largest organ for the manufacture of lymphocytes close to the small intestine. This organ is the spleen, whose function it is to send armies of lymphocytes to the villi after the ingestion of a meal. As these lymphocytes course through the lymph channels of the villi they absorb amino acids, the digested form of protein. They are then circulated toward a large duct, the thoracic duct, which gives them a quick right-of-way to the subclavian vein into which the thoracic duct empties, just above the point where the secretion of the thyroid gland is discharged into the same vein.

Thus the lymphocytes are exposed to the iodine of the thyroid gland which "iodizes" their amino acids, thereby making cell growth and reproduction possible. The lymphocytes then circulate in the blood vessels or the lymph vessels, or under certain conditions take a cross cut right through the tissues to a needed spot. They are able to do this because they are endowed with what is called "ameboid" movement. After supplying food material to the body cells for nourishment and reproduction, the lymphocytes return to the spleen, where they either disintegrate or are sent on again to the villi to start another cycle.

If this explanation seems bizarre to my readers—especially my medical friends—let me say that I first put forth the idea for this treatment in an editorial which was published in the December, 1928, *Journal of Laboratory and Clinical Medicine*. Warren T. Vaughan, M.D., then editor-in-chief, commented: "Dr. Bieler's hypothesis is alluring. They say that there is nothing new under the sun, but I don't recall having seen this hypothesis anywhere before." I believe the hypothesis to be fact, substantiated by many experiments, observations, and successfully-treated cases since that time.

There are two stages in the life of the body when lymphocytes are needed in larger than "normal" amounts: the stages of growth and of repair. During the rapid growth of childhood and until the end of adolescence there occurs what is called the "lymphocytosis of childhood." During this period nature has supplied an extra lymphocyte-manufacturing center—the thymus, which atrophies after adolescence. Nature was thoughtful enough to place the thymus so near the thyroid that impregnation with iodine is a simple matter.

Another fascinating function of the lymphocytes is their ability to act as defense cells which assist in the repair of injuries. In pathology this is called the "small round cell infiltration," observed around all areas of inflammation or destruction of tissues. Interestingly enough, injured cells are repaired at a much faster rate than normal or uninjured body cells are nourished. When the repair is complete, the rate of growth returns to the normal level.

I believe that the repair and alteration of rate of growth is controlled by impulses from the "abdominal brain," or solar plexus, and that its orders are telegraphed through the nerves of the sympathetic system—all part of an automatic process insuring self-preservation. Many scientific experiments and observations substantiate this explanation. A young animal deprived of its thymus shows great retardation of growth. This is true to an even greater degree when the thyroid is extirpated or depleted due to goiterous states. Certain drugs, too, can cause degeneration of the lymphocytes, resulting in a state called leucopenia, during which nourishment of the body is subnormal as well as is the rate of growth and repair of tissues. Other drugs, the ill-fated Thalidomide, for example, can so depress thyroid secretion as to result in failure of fetal cells to reproduce and multiply; as a consequence, the baby is armless, legless or otherwise deformed. The other extreme—an oversaturation of the lymphocytes with amino acids and iodine—could, I believe, cause cancer, an abnormal growth of cells in the localized area, resulting in a neoplasm, or malignant new growth.

During digestion carbohydrates and complex sugars are reduced to simple glucose, which is absorbed by the blood vessels of the villi and burned directly in the muscles. The body receives its muscular energy and heat in this manner. Fats also are combustible, but they usually burn best in a carbohydrate flame. Unneeded fats are sent to various parts of the body to be stored—a physiological fact of life which saddens and worries overweight Americans. Fat, together with minerals and trace elements (vitamins) and carbohydrates, are of vital importance to life.

How you feel—whether you sing, sigh or sob—is based mainly on how your fueling system works. "You can't ignore the importance of a good digestion," remarked Joseph Conrad. "The joy of life ... depends on a sound stomach, whereas a bad digestion inclines one to skepticism, incredulity, breeds black fancies and thoughts of death." Every physician is familiar with the "black fancies" expressed by those who complain of digestive troubles. When their bodies are freed of the toxic load they carry, an almost magical change takes place in the patients I have treated.

The full picture of digestion is a large, complex canvas and can be covered only in broad strokes in these pages. But I have attempted, in this chapter, to stress the role played by the villi. Their vitality insures a healthy state of life and can be maintained only by the most careful consideration of the quantity and quality of food ingested. And since the body is, more or less, the product of the food fed it, altering body chemistry by diet is not only feasible but most desirable in disease states. By accepting good food material or by rejecting irritating food material (usually by vomiting or diarrhea), the small intestine serves as *the first line of the body's defense against harmful foods and poisons*.

Errors of diet, when slight, are not immediately noticeable; gross errors produce immediate penalties. Just how the body rejects improper food is shown in many cases from my files. At random, I have selected one, that of a man of forty-two. He attended a dinner at which a variety of Mexican food was served, topped off by pie à la mode. Since he had skipped lunch that day, he admitted he did full justice to the dinner. That night he suffered violent diarrhea..

This meant that his body was utilizing the first line of defense—a rapid elimination of the offensive mixture of foods. When I saw him, the bowel was inflamed by his dietary indiscretion and I prescribed bed rest and diluted milk and yeast as his only nourishment for the next forty-eight hours. He desired no other food and needed none. Drugs, I believe, would have complicated his original trouble. A complete recovery followed. "I brought that attack on by my own folly," he said, "and it won't happen again."

Drug manufacturers and Madison Avenue television-commercial writers seem to be obsessed with the digestive system. Drug-store shelves are lined with a fantastic array of patent medicines, pills and food supplements for digestive malfunctions. And Americans squander millions on these products. If they knew something of body chemistry, they would realize they could use "dietary medicine" instead of pills to cure their digestive disorders. Why take a pill of inorganic chemicals when these same chemicals can be obtained *organically* from food? The thirty- to thirty-two-foot alimentary canal, long-suffering in its battle to protect the body from harm, has an able ally in the liver. In the next chapter we will learn how this remarkable organ functions as *the second line of defense against disease*.

6

The Liver: Second Line of Defense Against Disease

If you had been living in ancient Babylon and became seriously ill your physician, who doubled as priest, would have asked you to breathe into a sheep's nose. He would then have slaughtered the sheep, taken a "reading" of the liver, and predicted the outcome of your illness. These civilized ancients believed that a "breathed-on" sheep's liver would not only register the nature of the disease but the prospects for recovery as well. Believed to be the seat of all vital functions, the liver was the obvious choice of the gods for revealing their intentions.

—WILLIAM D. SNIVELY, THE SEA WITHIN

The ancients respected the liver and believed it to be not only the soul's center but the most important organ in the body. Yet during later centuries the liver was unaccountably neglected by the medical profession. "Indeed," say Benjamin F. Miller, M.D., and Ruth Goode in *Man and His Body*, "as late as a generation ago writers of texts on the human body had little to say about it except that it provided bile for the digestion. Today, we once more recognize the liver as a most extraordinary organ . . . It is not romantic like the heart or deep and mysterious like the brain. Yet it has a number of claims to uniqueness: it is the body's master chemist, also the fuel storage and supply office, housekeeper, and poison control center. In its unspectacular way it is about as hard-working an organ as we have; if we choose to list them we could put down some five hundred separate functions that it performs."

Nature also respects this largest (it weighs up to three pounds) and most solid organ inside the body, giving the liver special protection by tucking it out of harm's way under the strong muscular diaphragm and the bony support of the lower ribs. It is a tremendously tough gland, able to rebuild its missing cells and to regenerate damaged ones. It will function with only one fifth or less of its whole; in cancer cases as much as 90 percent of the liver has been removed and months later the gland has grown to its original size, if the patient has survived the operation. Thus, it may be considered potentially immortal. Nevertheless, constant abuse in the shape of malnutrition, harmful drugs, poisons and infection does eventually wear it out.

Man's original food and environment were found in the jungle. Although he has come far in the last ten thousand years and his previous existence may have covered a million years or so, his abdomen still contains a liver of which the basic chemistry is that of the jungle man. With civilization came gradual changes in man's food and his eating habits. Food was cooked, food was salted and, later, processed and chemically treated. But man's liver didn't change. It remained the old pre-civilization model.

The liver, then, is the central chemical laboratory in the body as well as its most important detoxicator. It is so important that man can live only a few hours without it. For this reason surgeons are inclined to eye it warily and seldom touch it except for the removal of an occasional tumor, abscess or cyst. Anyone who has studied the liver extensively knows that its manifold activities are so complicated and numerous that one could lose oneself in its labyrinths. Let us then discuss only the role of the liver in what I call the body's *second line of defense against disease,* just as digestion is the first line. Because of the liver's importance to the whole organism I have devoted much time to studying it along original lines. And I discovered many hitherto unknown facets of its functions. This research has enabled me to prescribe diets for "liver-exhausted" patients—diets which have aided them in regaining health.

Of all the alkaline elements of the body, sodium is the most important. It is my belief that the liver is the storehouse of these elements, especially of sodium. It is the element found in greatest abundance and is the most needed in maintaining the body's acid-base balance. Sodium is found in every cell of the body; also, there are large concentrated sodium-storage centers to be used in case of emergency. These concentrated areas have a great buffer value; in addition, much acid and corrosive poison can be neutralized and stored in them, more or less temporarily. Among the important sodium-storage reservoirs are the muscles, brain and nerves, bone marrow, skin, gastric and intestinal mucosa, the kidneys and the liver, which is by far the most important; it is richest of all the organs in sodium, its chief chemical element. Therefore, as the largest storehouse of sodium the liver is clearly the body's *second line of defense*.

When the liver is depleted of sodium in order to neutralize its acids, its function may be so severely inhibited that illness results. Are you aware that if the liver could keep the blood stream clean by filtering out damaging poisons, man could live indefinitely, barring physical accidents? It is only when the liver's filtration ability is hindered that the poisons get beyond the liver and into the general blood circulation. Only then do the symptoms of disease occur. And that is why you must guard your liver so carefully.

If, then, sodium is so important to good health, how do we obtain it? How can we conserve it? Sodium, the body's vital element, is derived from the sodium compounds in the diet. The richest source is in the vegetable kingdom and the next best source is found in certain animal tissues, such as muscle and liver. "Well," you may say, "I don't care much for vegetables; I'll eat potatoes but I love meat, so I have nothing to fear." Unfortunately, that is not the answer.

In order to obtain the sodium value from the meats you enjoy, they must be eaten *raw*, or as near raw, as possible. To many people raw or very rare meat is unpalatable. Yet it is not hard to prove on the basis of simple urine tests in the laboratory that the more meat is *cooked*, the more putrefaction acids are found in the urine of the over-proteinized patient. This means that an individual who eats few vegetables and salads and much overcooked meat frequently has a sodium-starved liver.

After the digestion of any meal, all of the blood from the intestines circulates through the liver, entering it by way of the large portal vein which flows directly into it. The useful elements from the digested food are taken to the liver which (1) synthesizes new body tissues, (2) prepares fuel for oxidation, and energy, (3) stores excess nourishment for future use.

Toxins and other harmful substances are neutralized by the liver and eliminated by the excretory secretion of the liver. This secretion is called bile. Sometimes the power of the liver to neutralize these toxic substances completely is curtailed because of insufficient alkalinity. The bile is then released to the small intestine in a toxic state. During the coursing of this toxic bile through the small intestine, if it has not already caused enough nausea to be eliminated quickly by vomiting, much of the harmful material is reabsorbed. At the same time it may cause various degrees of intestinal inflammation.

The presence of toxic bile in the intestine can also upset its digestion of useful food, giving rise to products of toxic indigestion, gas formation and much abdominal pain. In some respects bile is comparable to urine. Normally, it is clear bright yellow, alkaline in reaction and non-irritating to the tissues which confine it. When pathological, it changes to darker colors, being most toxic when dark green or black, at which time it has an intense acid and corrosive action on adjacent tissues. This dark-green bile can do nothing but harm. Normal alkaline bile is non-corrosive and compatible with almost any food. But as the liver is gradually depleted of its sodium—leached out for the neutralization of toxins—the normal sodium salts of the bile acids are formed with greater difficulty. When the bile is entirely too irritating to be poured over the contents of the duodenum (the first portion of the small intestine into which the bile ducts drain), it is stored temporarily in the gall bladder, where it is gradually neutralized. But toxic, acid or corrosive bile is incompatible with many foods. Consequently it creates an inflammation of the liver, of the bile ducts, of the gall bladder and of the intestines. At times it is regurgitated into the stomach and, if toxic enough, vomited.

In the duodenum irritation from abnormal bile can result in bile burns which, in turn, cause unpleasant and frightening spasms. The victim hastens to a doctor who takes X-rays. These films show distortion of duodenal shadows, often diagnosed as ulcers. My own research reveals that possibly 99 percent of X-ray-diagnosed ulcers are, in reality, merely bile burn spasms. Just as baseball is our chief national pastime, so might we call these spasms the chief American disease. And it is for the relief of these unpleasant symptoms that the popular anti-acid pills, wafers, lozenges and powders are dispensed by the millions. Of course, it *is* possible for the corrosion from a bile burn to develop into an ulcer, but fortunately this rarely occurs. True gastric or duodenal ulcer is rather rare, and it is not difficult to diagnose if a previous case has been seen: hemorrhage is always present and blood is either vomited or passed in the stools.

When there is a too rapid drain of the liver's available sodium, the liver cells die. Scar tissue results, the terminal phases of which are the different types of cirrhosis, or scarring, of the liver. But before it produces symptoms which are obvious, a cirrhotic liver is already severely damaged.

Civilization, with its processed, concentrated and synthesized foods, is responsible for the enormous quantities of antacid remedies sold and consumed in the form of pills, candies and chewing gum—"remedies" that temporarily relieve distress while doing nothing to remove the cause.

An interesting case from my files which shows kidney as well as liver malfunction is that of a man who was sixty-one when I first began treating him. He had been bedfast with dropsy of the legs and abdomen for two years. His abdomen was enormous. His adrenal glands were strong and active. There were times when he became irrational. His urine had the consistency of thick, dark molasses, was loaded with pus, albumen, and casts. He voided constantly, in dribbles. His blood pressure was 210/110. This patient had great difficulty breathing, due mainly to the pressure against his diaphragm from the fluid in his abdomen (ascites).

But he was a tough man and determined to get well. Luckily, he was cared for twenty-four hours a day by a most loving and meticulous daughter. His dietary history disclosed that he had been a heavy starch and dessert eater. Pastries, cakes, cookies and sweets of some type were consumed with every meal except breakfast. Much against his will, his daughter began to "manage" him. He was placed on diluted fruit juices for several weeks. At his bedside I introduced a needle and drained his ascites, which filled a five-gallon washtub! When all of this ascitic fluid had drained, his abdominal wall was so flabby that it was possible to feel the bowels, liver and spleen. The liver was about the size of a large orange, hard and nodular, intensely cirrhotic.

In all my years of practice, I had never seen so desperately situated a patient recover. After three weeks, the edema of the legs had subsided, but the ascites gradually reaccumulated. His urine became light-colored, the albumen reduced to one-plus. The casts disappeared. He was given easily digestible proteins, cooked and raw vegetables and fruits, while starches and sweets were restricted. He rebelled, but in a few more weeks he was content to follow this regime. In six months he was albumen-free and able to spar with his grandsons. It was necessary to tap his abdomen once a month during the first year, and each time approximately five gallons of fluid was drained. At that time he began to do light jobs around the house and garden. The second year he was tapped every two months; the third year every three months, the tappings averaging one to two gallons. During the fourth year, tapping ceased to be necessary.

After the abdominal distention resulting from such a huge amount of ascites, his abdominal muscles were weak and I cautioned him about the possible development of an umbilical hernia. His general musculature at this time was superb, and I had never seen such a soft, resilient, moist and clear skin. But one day, even though wearing an abdominal support, he lifted too heavy a rock. Two days later I was called and found a strangulated umbilical hernia. Surgery followed, from which he made a rapid and complete recovery. It was unnecessary to remove any bowel, although about twenty-four inches of the small intestine had a dark-blue color. Today, twelve years after treatment was started, he works hard, tending two neighbors' yards in addition to his own. He is seventy-three, with no complaints and, phenomenally, his liver has regained normal size and the hardness has disappeared.

A simpler case from my files is that of a man, thirty-five, who complained of extreme weakness, vertigo, nausea, vomiting and loss of appetite. Laboratory tests disclosed he was suffering from liver toxemia. Despondent and unable to sleep, he was a sorry sight. He was put to bed for five days, given a short fast on diluted vegetable broth. At the end of that time the liver function was sufficiently restored so that he was able to assimilate proper food. It was pointed out to him, in giving him a diet, that food and nutrition are not the same thing. Man is nourished not by the food he eats but only in proportion to what he is able to digest and assimilate.

The liver, then, is the body's principal organ of detoxication; the chemical wizard which performs its chemical magic with quiet efficiency; the strainer through which is poured all that finds its way into the body before it enters the general circulation. As long as the liver function is intact, the blood stream remains pure. When it becomes impaired, the toxins enter the circulation and cause irritation, destruction and eventually death.

7

The Endocrine Glands: Third
Line of Defense
Against Disease

Life is largely a matter of chemistry.
—WILLIAM J. MAYO, M.D.

The liver's waste-disposal role is of utmost importance to good health. When it begins to fail as a blood filter, we may expect that toxic material will enter the general circulation. It is this toxic material in the general circulation which stimulates the endocrine glands—*third line of defense against disease*—to *overactivity* in a valiant attempt to help the body neutralize and eliminate the irritants resulting from improper digestion of proteins, sugars, starches and fats.

In order to understand just how the amazing endocrine glands act to defend the body against disease, we must know something of their structure and operation. These small bits of tissue, the glands of *internal secretion* or *ductless* glands, are called endocrine (in-pouring); they differ from the glands of *external secretion* (such as sweat or tear glands) because they secrete the characteristic substances they manufacture directly into the blood stream rather than pouring them out through a tube or duct. The characteristic substances secreted by the various endocrine glands are called hormones, also spoken of as "biochemical messengers" of the blood. Hormones, even in extremely tiny amounts, are unbelievably potent; they direct and regulate much of the subtle biochemistry of life.

Although there are others, the three glands we are concerned with here are (1) the adrenal glands, (2) the thyroid gland, (3) the pituitary gland.

The amazing thing about these extraordinarily powerful glands is that they are so tiny. The thryoid gland, the giant in size, weighs approximately one ounce; the parathyroids are so tiny that they are scarcely visible; the adrenal glands are about the size of a small lima bean; the pituitary is about half an inch long, yet it regulates the other glands as well as performing important functions of its own.

Tiny though these glands may be, their roles in both health and disease are enormous. As Dr. Lewellyn Barker of Johns Hopkins once summed them up: "Our stature, the kinds of faces we have, the length of our arms and legs, the shape of the pelvis, the color and consistency of the integument, the quantity and regional location of our subcutaneous fat, the amount and distribution of hair on our bodies, the tonicity of our muscles, the sound of the voice, the size of the larynx and the emotions to which our exterior gives expression, all depend, to a large extent, upon the degree of functioning, during the early development period, of the endocrine glands."

THE ADRENALS: GLANDS THAT MAKE OXIDATION (LIFE) POSSIBLE

There is, at present, no doubt that the adrenals are the most necessary glands for sustaining life and health. The adrenal glands lie just over the kidneys and are composed of two portions: an inner layer called the medulla and an outer layer called the cortex.

The cortex of the adrenal gland is an integral part of the sympathetic nervous system, which controls and regulates many of the conscious and unconscious functions of the body. Its numerous connections with the solar plexus have been thoroughly identified. At about the seventh month of fetal life, the adrenal glands are equal to the kidneys in size. At birth they are slightly smaller and during life they gradually diminish in size until, in the aged, they can hardly be distinguished at autopsy. It has been stated that life in man is impossible without the adrenal secretion in the blood stream. Indeed, we doctors recognize the sudden fatal collapse following a hemorrhage into the adrenals, and we know the creeping death of the patient with Addison's disease (chronic deterioration of the adrenals).

The chemistry of life itself depends upon the process of oxidation. The secretion of the adrenal glands is the hormone which makes oxidation in the body cells possible. The adrenal glands determine whether or not the fire shall burn. It would be assuming too much to think that all the physical and chemical functions of the adrenal glands have been discovered, but the more important functions which have been studied and recorded to date are as follows:

1. Control of oxidation of all body cells, regulating
   (a) Nerve energy (oxidation of phosphorus in the brain and nerve tissue)
   (b) Physical energy and heat (oxidation of carbon in the muscles)
   (c) Special organ function (oxidation in liver and kidneys)
   (d) Life of every body cell (impossible without oxidation)
2. Control of tone of
   (a) Voluntary muscles (bodily strength)
   (b) Heart muscles (circulation, blood pressure)
   (c) Involuntary muscle (peristalsis; uterine tone)
3. Control of the number of circulating blood cells, red and white
4. Control of blood clotting (probably also assisted by parathyroids)
5. Control of the degree of body immunity
6. Control of the rate of red cell sedimentation.

THE THYROID GLAND:
NATURE'S PACE SETTER

"Johnny has drive and energy like me," a mother will tell me proudly, "but Mary is slow and calm like her dad. Isn't it all a matter of glands, Doctor?"

Well, not precisely. There are other complex factors involved, but it is likely that the rate of metabolism in Mary differs from that of Johnny. And the gland responsible for the difference in making the body's cellular engines poke along or race dangerously fast is the thyroid or pace-setter gland. Situated at the base of the neck, just below the "Adam's apple," the butterfly-shaped thyroid gland consists of two separate lobes joined by an isthmus. Although it was named in 1656 (from the Greek, meaning "shield"), it is only during the last forty years that it has been intensively studied. In addition to facilitating cell reproduction, among its more important functions are regulation of the rate of the following:

Oxidation in all of the body tissues
Repair of damaged or diseased body tissues
Sugar liberation from the liver to the blood stream
The heart beat
Brain and special sense activity
Normal cell growth.

THE PITUITARY: THE MASTER GLAND

The Roman physician Galen (b. A.D. 130), who was one of antiquity's most famous physicians, had a strangely erroneous idea concerning the functioning of the pituitary. He believed this master gland acted as a filter through which impurities were discharged from the brain into the throat. For fifteen hundred years physicians accepted this curious error. Even today we don't know much about the working of the pituitary, and its complexity is such that in the labyrinths of this tiny half-inch gland, the most skilled endocrinologists lose their way. And although they may not know fully "what makes it tick," they still regard it as marvelous. Asked to choose the most important single power of the pituitary, they would be like children with noses pressed to a toyshop window.

Shaped like a cherry hanging on a stem, the pituitary is situated inside the skull at the base of the brain; it rests in a small bony cave called the *sella tursica* (Turkish saddle), located directly behind the eyeballs. As master, its special function is to trigger other members of the endocrine system to get busy and produce their particular hormones. It is divided into three parts. The anterior portion, with a distinctly glandular function, discharges its secretion into the blood stream. This hormone probably:

(1) Determines the size and stature of the body
(2) Determines the degree of intelligence and higher cortical activity
(3) In a manner not wholly understood at present, controls the sex function.

The central portion of the pituitary gland contains the intermediate canals, lined with special nerve cells fringed with cilia, which wave in the passing blood stream and can test the chemistry of the blood. This same organ is highly developed in certain fishes —our remote ancestors—for determining the chemistry of the sea water. In a like manner this test organ in man's pituitary detects foreign toxins in the blood stream and alerts a defense mechanism to act against them.

The posterior portion of the pituitary, rich in highly specialized nerve cells, is really a part of the brain itself—a tiny segment which dips down into this location. Its cells are rich in hormones, which stimulate the sympathetic nervous system and through this stimulation cause increase of tone and strength of contraction of the smooth muscles.

So we have seen something of the workings of three of the endocrine glands. But just how do they act as the third line of defense against disease?

In order to understand this function we must return to the pituitary gland, well called both the body's "watchdog" as well as its central "telegraph office." This tiny but powerful master gland is the size of the tip of a little finger. Nevertheless, it is of incalculable importance to man's well-being. Nature wisely provided protection when she situated the pituitary deep within the skull. Life itself ebbs, if the tiny pituitary gland fails, because it is the pituitary that secretes a large number of the most important hormones.

The middle section of the pituitary is rich in blood vessels, lined with nerve cells fringed with long streamers, or cilia. The cilia are detectors which test the chemistry of the circulating blood. When toxins are present in the passing current of blood, a signal is given which eventually travels to the thyroid and adrenal glands, which with the pituitary gland constitute a *third line of defense against disease.*

During an emergency the pituitary signals the thyroid and adrenal glands to begin directing elimination of the toxic material from the blood. The thyroid and adrenals respond by directing the toxins into the only paths they are able to. *In emergencies the thyroid will direct elimination through the skin and the mucous and serous membranes; the adrenals will direct elimination through the kidneys and bowels.*

An example to illustrate this sort of diseased condition resulting from elimination of highly concentrated toxins is a bronchitis of the lungs, which is a catarrhal exudation through the mucous membrane lining the bronchial tubes. The violent cough characteristic of this disease is nature's attempt to expel the exudative toxic material. The lungs remain inflamed following such a crisis for several days. It is after this type of vicarious elimination that the patient enjoys an improved state of health, until the concentration of toxins is built up again.

You have all seen people whose faces and throats showed evidence of goiter. A patient of mine, a woman of fifty-eight, showed such evidence. She complained of great weakness, sweating, racing heart, protruding eyes and swelling of the legs. A classic type of exophthalmic goiter, her thyroid gland had been overstimulated by an existing toxemia. Here, again, the cure is effected by neutralizing the toxemia. Cases such as this are difficult to cure and require long bed rest. Due to the overactive thyroid, which accelerates catabolism, they must be fed this neutralizing diet while resting. The character of the diet will depend on the condition of the patient and his ability to digest. In this case, the patient was put to bed for six weeks and the diet consisted of raw milk and cooked and raw non-starchy vegetables. The amount of milk was determined by the daily condition of the patient. A complete recovery followed.

A case I am presently treating, that of a forty-four-year-old man, is also responding to treatment. For some eight months before I first saw him, he scarcely had been able to sleep because of the overactivity of his thyroid gland, which was "pinch-hitting" for the liver. He was deeply upset. After only four days on a vegetable broth fast, he began to be able to sleep; gradually the distressing symptoms of hyperthyroidism are subsiding.

Let me stress again that the path of the eliminated toxins will depend largely upon the comparative and potential strength of the endocrine glands. Should the thyroid be the strongest, we would expect the vicarious elimination to take place through the skin, either through the outside skin (the hide), the inside skin (mucous membranes), or the middle skin (serous membranes). Should the adrenals predominate, vicarious elimination may occur through the bowels or the kidneys, or the toxic materials literally could be burned up by hyperoxidation in the liver, effected by adrenal response, often giving rise to elevated body temperature or fever.

The potential strength of the glands of internal secretion depends upon two main factors: heredity and the state of the glands following chemical (dietetic) and emotional disturbances. Whichever gland has the greatest potential strength at the time of crisis will determine the avenue of vicarious elimination. But it must be pointed out that *too frequent use* of the same paths of vicarious elimination will lead to atrophy and degeneration of any path of elimination as well as a gradual wearing down of the strength of the glands themselves.

When man does not overstep nature's limits regarding harmful diet and emotional indulgences, the liver, as I mentioned earlier, acting as a second line of defense, is able to keep the general circulation pure. Under such utopian conditions, it is conceivable that disease would be an impossibility. In other words, the individual, under these circumstances, would be immune to disease.

8

You—Under the Doctor's Eye

> The widely held supposition that physique is irrelevant to behavior and personality is downright nonsense. Your carcass is the clue to your character.
>
> —EARNEST A. HOOTON, PH.D.

Into my office daily come patients with every conceivable type of physique and temperament. To an experienced physician's eye, the appearance of the new patient offers a good many clues to his state of health before a word of his medical history is taken. Each patient carries an indefinable something that differentiates him from another individual. Biochemically, too, our bodies are individual. The proteins that are peculiarly our own have no exact duplicates; they, as well as our tissues, cells and blood, are modified by heredity, disease states, blood constituents and a host of other factors. So each individual's inner environment differs radically from the next one. And his reactions, therefore, to his outer environment are just as different.

Doctors have always sought some method of classification of patients in order to make treatment easier. Yet there are many overworked doctors who like to hand out printed "low-caloric diets" to all their obese patients, even though they know that each patient varies from the next. I am frequently approached by medical colleagues who hear of my experience with diet in the treatment of various diseases: "Please give me your migraine diet." "I understand you have an arthritis diet that works. What is it?" "What do you feed diabetics to enable them to give up insulin?" "What special foods do you recommend for ulcer, hypertension, cancer, etc., etc.?"

In each case my answer is, "There is no *one* diet for this disease that you can print up and hand out. Show me the patient and let me examine him; then I can formulate a diet for his *specific* condition." Offhand diet-making would be as unscientific as relying on the blanket diets of the so-called nutritionists, who attribute magic qualities to the "food myths" they sell at high prices.

Patients and friends always ask me what I eat, so they can attempt to duplicate my own energy, my mountain climbing, my daily work load and love of life at an advanced age. Certainly I have no arcane secrets. But I cannot, in all honesty, be as specific as they would like. As an individual I differ profoundly from others; as a physician I try to go beyond the visible disease. I must distinguish the disease in the patient from the disease described in the medical books. The patient I am treating must be exhaustively studied, his condition recognized. If possible, he must be relieved of his symptoms and cured.

That is why this book must remain general. It is not a recipe for getting well. All formulas, diets, instructions must be general. Medicine can never be practiced from a book but only from a careful study of the patient, laboratory tests, and so on. After I have studied and talked with the patient and made the tests, I determine whether or not his body is toxic. If it is, I prescribe a special diet to cleanse the system; then a building-up of the patient is in order and this can be accomplished in many different ways, depending on his physical condition and the nature of his toxemia. To cure him I must study him as an individual, note his resistance to various factors, understand the life he leads today and the life he led in the past. He is an individual and his treatment must therefore be unique. I cannot try, as a clothing salesman might, to fit a stock-size coat to individuals of different shapes.

A good example of the complexity of the human body is the number of amino acids, or building blocks, it contains, all of which are obtained from protein in the diet. In a dictionary are many thousands of words, all built up from the twenty-six letters of the alphabet. Similarly, protein is made from millions of different combinations of amino acids, of which there are more than two dozen. A keen-nosed dog can identify his master among hundreds of individuals and the mother seal can find her pup amid thousands of similar-looking baby seals. So, no one man's protein can really resemble in odor or taste the protein in another individual's tissues. In addition, his body is modified by the diseases and drugs he has had, by his heredity and by other factors. That is why individuals react differently to disease, to drugs and to diet. Because of this very individuality, one cannot write a book on how to cure various diseases. Still, there are physicians who have written such books. Most of these writers are circumscribed by their own horizons: the doctor who was ill and regained his health on a diet of carrots, for example, believes he can save the world by making a "carrot diet" a way of life.

While it is true that each patient in a doctor's office is unique, in one way all patients are quite similar: they do not consult a doctor until illness strikes. Primarily, they want *relief:* relief from pain, relief from insomnia, relief from indigestion. And the doctor is supposed to give them relief and to give it quickly. Unfortunately, there is no way to give "instant relief" except through stimulation or depression. And that treatment is the result of whipping or paralyzing the endocrine glands, most usually the adrenal glands, which produce a temporary *effect* of well-being. Stimulation or depression is not health. Sleeping pills at night, pep pills in the morning, tranquilizers during the day—this is not health. And health is what I believe the conscientious physician truly should strive to achieve.

In a sense patients themselves are to blame for this method of therapy. They want to feel well, to be relieved immediately of pains which aggravate them; they want to be able to get through the day somehow and to sleep more or less soundly at night. They are not really interested in overall health, and if the doctor practices in another fashion—if he explains to the sufferer that his body chemistry is faulty, that before he will be permanently free of his symptoms his whole chemistry will have to be changed—the patient quickly becomes impatient. Cleansing a body of its metabolic poisons is a slow process. People gorge themselves over a long period of time, then expect the doctor to make them sylphlike in a few weeks.

Most ill persons are not very much interested in long-term treatment because they still believe so firmly in superstition, miracle drugs and the knife. They are not interested in experiencing really radiant health. What they are after, as I have indicated, is instant cessation of their symptoms. Or, as Madison Avenue has it: "Feel better faster." And if the doctor doesn't give it to them, the drug store will. Or they begin shopping around for another doctor, not realizing that regaining health is a long process, one that might take a whole year or longer. Yet they understand that when an individual suffers from advanced tuberculosis, it usually means years of rest in a sanitarium.

Every doctor knows that people tend to suppress awareness of disease. "The reason for such opposition," according to Dr. Ian Stevenson, is that "disease begins for the most part as a slight deviation from normal function. But the average person is too engrossed in his own purposes to be concerned with the normality of his functions. Illness to him is not a departure from healthful living but an interference with the routine pleasures of life. He will recognize the existence of disease only when he becomes aware of symptoms which clamorously intrude on the pattern of his daily business. Even then he may belittle the idea that there is anything seriously the matter with him, and the admission may frequently be postponed until the scene is more fittingly dominated by a clergyman than by a physician. In this way, much time passes between the cessation of what we consider health and the evidence of what we do consider disease."

Many patients came to me because they were disappointed in the orthodox handling of their maladies. They came especially for dietary reform, because they suspected that food had a good deal to do with their disorders and their symptoms. They were predisposed, then, to follow some dietary advice. Unless a person has knowledge of the buoyant bodily health, mental clarity and abundant energy to be attained by improving his selection of food, he is apt to lack motivation to change old food habits for new ones. Once committed to small portions of lightly broiled lean meats, large servings of steamed vegetables, fresh fruits and green salads, whole-grain bread and certified raw milk, he is amazed at the change in his health. And when his palate is re-educated to appreciate the subtle flavor in these foods, he will not miss the stimulation obtained by dousing them with salt, pepper, catsup, vinegar or mustard and washing them down with sweetened cola drinks or coffee and tea.

I have found that most people have a hazy conception of diet—more hazy, if possible, than the average doctor, and the doctor's conception of diet is hazy enough. I find that I must explain these matters very carefully to a patient. I show him a picture of the inside of the liver; I describe the functions of that important organ and the other endocrine glands and I find that most people are fascinated by this knowledge. It makes the patient more co-operative, gives him a sense of participating in his own cure, largely because I stress the fact *that he must cure himself*; I cannot do any more than help him adjust himself to his particular type of food and treatment. I point out to him that once his body is cured of its toxemia, he will not have to remain on so rigid a diet as he needs while he is getting rid of the toxemia. The cure comes from within. Nature effects it; the physician is only a collaborator with nature, guiding his patient through the sometimes mystifying steps necessary to the handling of his specific problem.

When a sick person enters the doctor's office for the first time, he does not realize that his very appearance offers clues to his illness, his patterns of behavior, what organic diseases are likely to affect him and how time will deal with him. And that brings me to the subject of body-typing.

Each newborn baby is unique; among the billions of human beings there is not one other with that baby's variations of genes and of anatomy, which are beyond computation. And because of those tremendous individual differences, we have a Lincoln and a Hitler, a Gandhi and a Jack-the-Ripper. People may also react in the *same* manner because they belong to the same constitutional type.

Doctors in ancient times used a system of classification based on the individual's form (thin or fat) or according to his temperament (choleric, phlegmatic, sanguineous, melancholic—terms we still use today). Hippocrates divided man into classifications according to blood, phlegm and the color of the bile, and told his students they must observe body structure in order to make accurate diagnoses.

Many medical observers have devised various systems of using body build—"somatotyping"—in a hopeful attempt to fit all men into tight little categories. Dr. William H. Sheldon, in his exhaustive *Atlas of Men,* correlated the body types into three overall classes: the fleshy endomorphs; the muscular mesomorphs; and the thin ectomorphs. But this classification does not tell us much about the individual differences—differences we obtain from the huge grab-bag of genes from which each person receives a unique assortment.

It remained for a rather new science—endocrinology (from two Greek words, "within" and "separate")—to give us a new method of classifying human beings. The ancients made groping attempts to understand the functions of the important endocrine glands. But only after painstaking work over the last fifty years has endocrinology begun to unlock its mysteries. And since the endocrine secretions—called hormones, from the Greek "to arouse"—actually determine the physical and neurological types of individuals, it naturally follows that endocrinology offers us the best approach to typing them.

Though much of the endocrine system still remains hidden, we do know that individuals can be grouped according to the internal secretions which control their development. Individuals and families, even races and nations, show definite internal secretion traits which stamp them with particular racial, national, family and individual qualities—physical characteristics that differentiate them from others.

We know that many mysterious body conditions are caused by endocrine imbalance. But a good part of the medical profession, unfortunately, has been equally mystified as to how to treat a number of those imbalances. There has been a sad loss of interest in endocrinology by these doctors, because the therapeutic value of the endocrines disappointed them. Vitality depends upon sound activity of the endocrine glands, for they discharge powerful hormones and act as a stimulus on living cells. If a patient's adrenal or thyroid glands were weak, they reasoned, then all one had to do would be to administer some adrenal or thyroid extract. When the extracts failed to accomplish the hoped-for results, these medical men lost interest in endocrinology. They completely disregarded the largest endocrine gland of the body, the liver, and failed to realize that many of the disturbances of the endocrine glands will clear up if an unhealthy liver is brought back to normal function.

As the science of endocrinology advanced it was found that the endocrine glands were responsible for such abnormalities as giants, dwarfs, cretins (stunted, deformed and mentally deficient), myxedematous individuals (grossly deficient in thyroid function), acromegalics (characterized by gigantism, enlarged head, feet, etc.) and various types of obesity. Much was learned from studies of the effects of removal of certain endocrine glands from animals in the laboratory. Also revealed were changes in growth and temperament resulting from overstimulation of the various endocrine glands. Most important of all, it became possible to predict and understand the cause and progress of many diseases characterized by symptoms due to endocrinologically-controlled avenues of vicarious elimination.

In order to aid in the diagnosis and treatment of disease, endocrinology has paved the way by classifying individuals into classic gland types: adrenal; thyroid; pituitary.

THE TYPICAL ADRENAL TYPE

Most of the information concerning the characteristics of the adrenal type of person has been the result of four sources of study: patients suffering from Addison's disease; adrenalectomized animals and human beings; the selective breeding of animals; patients with adrenal tumors. Among the animals, through careful breeding to augment adrenal strength, the draft horse, the shorthorn bull and the bulldog are examples which tend to confirm observations made upon man.

Physical examination of the typical adrenal type shows the following characteristics:

HAIR:	Of head—coarse and often curly; of body—coarse and thick, often characterized by a "hairy ape" appearance
FEATURES:	Coarse, large and heavy
EYES:	The iris shows ample pigmentation, either dark blue, brown or black; the pupil is small and reacts instantly
FOREHEAD:	Low, usually with a low hair line
NOSE:	Well developed, with large nostrils
LIPS:	Full, slightly negroid, with strong color and warmth, due to ample circulation
TEETH:	Large, especially the canines, yellowish in color, extremely hard and resistant to caries; the dental arches are full and round; the third molars usually erupt normally
TONGUE:	Thick, wide and clean; papillae coarse and thick
PALATE:	Low-arched and wide
SKULL:	Wide across the temples. Lower jaw heavy, solid and often protruding
EARS:	The lobe thick, large and long
SKIN:	Thick; dry and warm
NECK:	Thick and short; the characteristic "bull" type
CHEST:	Broad and thick, containing large heart and lungs
ABDOMEN:	Wide, thick and often protuberant
GENITALS:	Large
EXTREMITIES:	Thick and short; fingers and toes stubby; nails short, thick and with moons small or lacking

The physical energy of the adrenal type is seemingly inexhaustible, as is the nervous response of the sympathetic system, a result of perfect oxidation of phosphorus in the nerve tissue. Oxidation of carbon in the muscular system gives the adrenal type his great warmth. Thus, the temperature of his body is scarcely ever below 98.8, with hands and feet always pleasantly warm. As digestion and detoxication of food poisons depend greatly upon oxidation in the liver and intestines, it follows that the typical adrenal type, with his perfect oxidation, has thorough digestion. In fact, he may and often does boast that he can eat any and all kinds of food without discomfort. The exogenous uric acid products as well as the indoxyl compounds are completely detoxicated in the liver, do not accumulate in the blood, nor are they found in the urine.

The skeletal muscles are well developed and have splendid tone. Fatigue is practically unknown to the adrenal type. His muscular endurance is spectacular. And the perfect tone of the involuntary muscles is evidenced by complete and rapid peristalsis, resulting in several bowel evacuations daily. He can dine on the most impossible food combinations imaginable with no evil results, because his stomach muscles operate so well that some foods can be sidetracked while other foods are switched into the small intestine. This faculty has been corroborated by X-ray studies and by gastric lavage. A pregnant adrenal-type woman generally goes through her labor quickly, often having just one long, steady pain.

The quality of the blood is characteristic. A slight to marked polycythemia (more red cells than usual) occurs; leucopenia, or abnormal white cell count on the low side, is never noted. The blood, which is of a rich, red color, clots quickly. Fatal hemorrhage ·seldom occurs. The immunity against bacterial invasion is spectacular. The typical adrenal type hardly ever becomes infected, even with venereal diseases. The red cell sedimentation rate is slower than the so-called normal; often there is no apparent settling of the red corpuscles during the first hour of the test.

·A member of the adrenal-type group has a phlegmatic disposition —easygoing, jolly, slow to anger, never bothered with insomnia, fear or "cold feet." He will often go out of his way to avoid a quarrel.

Customarily, he has a wide circle of friends because he is warm-hearted and surrounded by an "aura" of kindly sympathy.

Splendid circulation gives him warm, magnetic hands, hence success as a masseur and magnetic healer. This warm-handed, warm-hearted adrenal type makes an excellent doctor, but unfortunately he is not often intelligent enough to meet entrance requirements for medical college. And, as a result, if he is sufficiently motivated, he will end up as an "irregular" doctor or healer. A strong adrenal type who is also fortunate enough to possess "brains," that is, a good pituitary gland, frequently becomes the most successful doctor of all.

Since members of this group have great muscular strength, patience, together with an I.Q. in the lower range, they make up the peasant-worker class or the unskilled-labor group.

THE TYPICAL THYROID TYPE

Physical examination of the thyroid type of individual shows the following characteristics:

HAIR: Of head—fine and silky; of body (except on pubis and in axillae)—hardly noticeable because it is so fine and thinly distributed

FEATURES: Delicate and finely molded; great beauty is the rule

EYES: Large and often slightly prominent—the type called "soulful"

TEETH: Narrowly spaced, of moderate size; pearly white, soft and not resistant to caries; dental arches usually V-shaped rather than round; partially erupted or unerupted third molars

TONGUE: Moderately thin and long, with fine papillae and sensitivity

PALATE: High; more V-shaped than arched

NECK: Graceful, thin and long

CHEST: Long and thin; heart usually smaller than so-called normal; exquisitely-shaped breasts in female; nipples more sensitive than in adrenal types .

ABDOMEN: Long and usually thin

GENITALS: Medium in size; their increased sensitivity makes up for their lack of size

EXTREMI-   Finely molded, graceful hands; beautiful fingers,
TIES: shapely, neither stubby nor markedly elongated

The most remarkable characteristic of the thyroid individual is his high-strung and extremely sensitive nervous system. He is the classic "race-horse" type, just as the adrenal person is the "draft horse" type. Thin, wiry, restless, quick, always on the jump, always listening, watching, smelling, because all the special senses of the thyroid person are highly developed. The heart beat is usually above 72 and the least shock to his nervous system will result in an accelerated pulse.

Simultaneous with cardiac acceleration is an increased secretion from the salivary and intestinal glands, liver, kidneys and sweat glands. The liver discharges sugar from the blood stream more rapidly and if the pancreatic function which maintains the concentration of blood sugar is weak, glycosuria (sugar in the urine) follows. Due to an increased metabolic rate, the body is likely, literally, to burn up and lose weight. The cerebration of the thyroid individual is most interesting. Usually several streams of thought actually whirl through his brain at once, making concentration most difficult. He is frequently fatigued, dissatisfied with his surroundings, home, friends and work.

In the adrenal type, it was noted that the adrenals determined whether or not the fire (oxidation) shall burn. The thyroid gland says how *fast* the fire shall burn.

Female members of the thyroid group, especially when the gland is overstimulated, find their menstrual cycle shortened, sometimes from twenty-eight to fourteen days. Their period of gestation is also shortened, from 280 days to 270 days or less. Generally, their babies are small and thin but usually healthy. The thyroid regulates the flow of breast milk, and it is the thin, wiry types that have breast milk to spare.

Typically, the thyroid gland types suffer from insomnia, restlessness and when they finally do fall asleep, they dream a great deal, with nightmares prevailing. Still, they awaken early, apparently fresh and with the day's plans formulated. Their sexual sensations are exquisitely developed. Orgasms, rapidly induced and frequently repeated, are accompanied with great intensity of feeling.

THE TYPICAL PITUITARY TYPE

HEAD:	Large, the skull high and often dome-like; the frontal bone and superior orbital ridges often prominent
FEATURES:	The upper lip is usually longer than normal
TEETH:	Usually large, especially the central incisors
JOINTS:	Laxity of all joints; knock knees and flat feet are common
EXTREMI-TIES:	Legs and arms long, which gives the tallness so commonly found in this type of person; fingers long and thin with large moons on the nails

The chart of the pituitary type is less complete than the other two types because research is limited at present. Although it is more difficult to discuss the pituitary type of individual because conclusions, to date, are based upon conjectural hypotheses, it is fairly agreed by the medical profession that oversecretion of the anterior pituitary may cause giants or acromegalics and that lack of this same secretion may result in dwarfism. It is estimated that some ten thousand individuals in the United States are considered dwarfs because they lack this essential growth hormone.

There is also an understanding of how the enlarged anterior pituitary can press against the side walls of the *sella tursica*, causing various degrees and kinds of headaches, and how the pressure can be exerted toward the optic chiasm (the crossing of the optic nerves just behind the eyeballs), resulting in diminution of the visual fields and perhaps total blindness. There is even weighty evidence that a sudden swelling of an anterior pituitary gland restricted by a less roomy, ricket-deformed *sella tursica* can result in convulsions characteristic of epilepsy. But of the true effect of the anterior pituitary on what may be termed higher brain functions, little is known. It is believed that the pituitary type is richer in "soul qualities"—intuition, creative ability, poetic expression, artistic temperament—and that his sexual drive is strongly developed.

As the reader attempts to fit himself into any of the above types, he will probably find that he does not wholly belong in any one category—he spills over. As Dr. Sheldon pointed out, the individual will always defy the statistics. Most of us are a combination of the three basic classic gland types. But one type is always dominant and that one is the key to our physical and mental profiles. We are all aware that we belong either to the "morning people" who arise ready to conquer the world or to the "night people" who come alive late in the day and we know that these varying metabolic patterns play havoc in marital relations—if we let them. Using the clues to personality and physique under discussion, we can do some important detective work on ourselves. For "know thyself" has ever been the philosopher's first maxim.

Since the so-called well-rounded individual cannot be strictly classified under any one of the glandular types, there is a method for determining which of the glands is truly dominant. For example, if the number 100 is taken for the normal value of any gland, then the normal person's pituitary, adrenals and thyroid all would be 100. His glandular equation would be:

Pituitary   100
Thyroid   100
Adrenals   100

But the pituitary type would always be deficient in either thyroid or adrenals and thus might have an equation such as:

Pituitary   150
Thyroid   50
Adrenals   100

This equation might well represent the lazy, impractical dreamer. But if we find Pituitary 150, Thyroid 100 and Adrenals 50, we have

the individual known as a genius. Because of the highly gifted
individual's subnormal adrenals, it is necessary for him to be constantly stimulating them, which he does by excessive use of food
stimulants such as meat, coffee, tea and salt, or he resorts to alcohol,
perhaps to narcotic drugs. When he has succeeded in lashing his
adrenals to 100-percent activity, his pituitary and thyroid become
overstimulated so that his equation would read as follows:

Pituitary	200
Thyroid	150
Adrenals	100

In this state he would have the most intense desire to work, to
create a perfect piece of art. The result could, and has been, a
masterpiece—a symphony, a poem, a painting or sculpture, a heroic
piece of literature. Following the period of overstimulation comes
the inevitable depression, during which time he is unable to create
anything at all—truly a suicidal state. If these periods of depression
did not occur and the flames of artistic creation were kept blazing,
sooner or later the adrenals would become entirely worn out, with
a tragic, too-early death the result.

Few of us are "geniuses," fortunately or not, depending on our
goals in life, but all of us want to understand the kind of people we
are and to fathom, too, the baffling differences among our relatives
and friends. But a doctor who understands it may use glandular
typing to determine whether we live long or short lives and whether
or not we might get specific diseases.

A dramatic case from my files will serve to illustrate how I use
observation of "body build" and the science of endocrinology (in
addition to routine laboratory tests) to gain an understanding of
an individual's illness; a clue to how his endocrine imbalance may
be restored; a knowledge of what paths his vicarious elimination
will take; what foods to use for his cure; finally, what diet to prescribe to keep him in good health thereafter. Without this knowledge of his body type and the state of his endocrine system, I would
be groping in the dark instead of proceeding on a well-defined path.

One morning an extremely worried woman helped her husband

into my office. Mr. L. was very weak, short of breath and he could scarcely move as he tried desperately to place one foot ahead of the other. The exertion left his face beet-red. I immediately helped him onto an examining table so that he could rest and begin to breathe more normally. He told me that his wife had driven him down from their home in Pasadena to my office in Capistrano Beach, a distance of sixty-five miles.

Mr. L. was the head of a huge company which printed Western editions of some twenty-six magazines and employed eleven hundred people. He told me he had been in excellent health until a year previously. When he became ill, he was placed under the care of a group of eighteen prominent Pasadena specialists, who had tried unsuccessfully to treat him at the Huntington Memorial Hospital for some four months.

His first symptom was a conjunctivitis, which turned his eyes blood-red. Then he developed pneumonia, for which he was given a shot of aureomycin. The next day he developed small inflamed areas in the mouth resembling canker sores, and these gradually increased in size until his mouth, lips and throat were a mass of reddened, inflamed tissue. There was much local pain, weakness and shortness of breath. At this point he was taken to the Huntington Hospital where a consultation was called. The doctors could not agree whether the diagnosis was *erythema multiforme* or *pemphigus*. A four-month treatment with intravenous ACTH eased his throat pain and enabled him to swallow more comfortably; during this time he was given the drug for eight hours daily. Soon he developed acute cardiac fibrillation (a violent fluttering of the heart). His physicians then changed the treatment and he was given cortisone hypodermically and later orally in pill form. The dosage was pushed to the point at which deformation occurs and soon the patient developed the syndrome of Cushing's disease, characterized by moon face and buffalo hump. Unhappily, there was little or no response to this therapy. His antibiotic bill amounted to about $1,500. Other therapies were added and one day he was given over $350 worth of gamma globulin. At this juncture his doctors agreed that he was not responding to treatment, and that the prognosis was extremely serious. At the same time his eye specialist predicted that he would be blind in three months.

This, then, was the problem lying on my examining table that morning.

Examination disclosed a tall, well-developed, muscular man in his late fifties. His face was plethoric, overloaded with fluids, his eyes were fiery red, his lips, mouth and throat were covered with sores. There was much pain and he could scarcely swallow. As I studied him for his gland type, I paid particular attention to his earlobes, which were thick, large and well-formed—a characteristic of the adrenal type. This also gave me a clue as to the functioning of his liver. Such study led me to suspect that he would have a chance to get well if I could improve his liver function and neutralize his toxemia. His thyroid gland and his pituitary gland were also valiantly trying to pinch-hit for the liver.

The amount of plethora in his body was enormous; his circulation seemed to be overwhelmed by an excess of red blood cells which apparently were not able to carry oxygen to the tissues. The saturation of these cells with drugs made them not only unable to carry oxygen but added to their weight. When he stood up, these cells would settle in his legs causing them to become blue-black in color. Examination of his liver disclosed that it was enlarged and showed a state of chronic passive congestion. The vein pressure was elevated and the plethora test applied to the skin of his back indicated that the corticoids were whipping his heart in an effort to neutralize the intense vein pressure. I decided that the toxemia from drugs was his most serious complication and would have to be relieved before his secondary toxemia (which caused the mouth lesions) could be treated.

These lesions were the result of a vicarious elimination through the mucous membranes of his lips, throat and mouth. This avenue of elimination was under the control of the thyroid gland, which was overcompensating. The adrenals, stimulated by the corticoids, were forcing toxins through the kidneys, bowels and liver. Thus, the adrenal glands, by elevating the blood pressure, managed to meet the increased vein pressure which otherwise would have dilated his heart and caused death.

"Your ultimate recovery depends on your body's ability to eliminate its toxemia—compósed of the drugs given you and of dietetic poisons," I told Mr. L. "First we will attempt to relieve the strain on the liver. Your liver has been forced to overexert itself. In order to give it as much rest as possible you must remain in bed and fast on small amounts of a special vegetable soup. All the useless red blood cells which have overwhelmed your circulation will have to be destroyed and their poisons eliminated from your body. This has been such a burden on the liver and spleen that the proper digestion and assimilation of food has been impossible. That is why I am fasting you on the vegetable soup. Gradually I expect to see evidence of a reduction in the toxemia, determined by urine and stool examination."

"Will I stop taking the drugs?" he asked.

"No," I told him. "During this time, no reduction in the drug dosage is possible because of the danger to your heart."

In a short time we were gratified to see much alleviation of his most distressing symptoms. After a month, fruit and fruit juices were added to his diet and fresh goat's milk in teaspoonful doses was tried. Mr. L. was extremely co-operative; his formerly hopeless outlook and fears for his recovery disappeared as he began to feel better.

Now I felt was the time to try to reduce the dosage of corticoids. Week by week the dose was decreased infinitesimally while I carefully observed the balance of his heart. This is an extremely delicate and dangerous procedure in a man as sick as this patient was, because as the heart becomes less stimulated, the adrenals are also less stimulated by the corticoids. Unless the vein pressure, in direct ratio, had been lowered by improvement in the liver congestion, an imbalance of the arterial-venous pressure could easily have been fatal. The withdrawal of the drugs consequently took many months and for several weeks after they were discontinued the patient was carefully observed at four-hour intervals. By this time the moon face and buffalo hump had disappeared. Increasing amounts of fruit and vegetables were given and about eight ounces daily of fresh goat's milk, in intervals, was well tolerated. Naturally, his recovery was a slow affair. It took eleven months for the acidity and dark color of the urine as well as the fetid odor of the stools to disappear.

A diet was gradually evolved which consisted of the following:

BREAKFAST:	One shredded wheat biscuit
	Four ounces of raw goat's milk
	Four stewed prunes
FORENOON:	Eight ounces of raw goat's milk
NOON AND NIGHT:	Six ounces of vegetable soup
	One pound of cooked string beans
	One piece of white bread with butter
	Eight ounces of raw goat's milk
AFTERNOON:	Eight ounces of raw goat's milk.

On this diet his recovery was complete. There were no more sores in his mouth; his eyesight is better than it has been for years; he can drive a golf ball farther than he ever could and there is no manual work about his home which he cannot do, including climbing ladders and repairing the roof.

Examination shows his heart, blood pressure and endocrine balance as well as the chemistry of the urine and bile to be perfectly normal. The liver function is also perfect and there is no sign of plethora, nor has there been any pathology since he recovered under my care five years ago. He still continues his careful diet.

The physician who is well grounded in endocrinology can often predict the course and outcome of a disease. As he goes through the wards of a hospital filled with patients suffering from tuberculosis, to cite one example where gland types are particularly noticeable, he easily recognizes three general types of individuals, as follows.

First, there is the thin, wiry *thyroid type* whose glandular equation is Pituitary 75, Thyroid 100, Adrenals 50 (this means that his pituitary gland is impaired to the extent of 25 percent; the thyroid normal; the adrenals only developing half of their functional capacity). Since the pituitary and adrenal glands are subnormal, the 100-percent thyroid tends to exaggerate the thyroid characteristics. Therefore, this patient is high-strung, nervous, always changing his mind—and his doctor—and is never satisfied with the hospital food or care he is receiving; he is troubled with gas, indigestion and constipation. Need I add that he constitutes a trial for the physician in charge?

In spite of forced feeding, it is impossible to put flesh on his bones; in fact, he often loses weight so rapidly that his gaunt appearance becomes alarming. He is the champion "night sweater"— of the drenching variety. When cavities develop in his lungs, they increase in size in spite of treatment. Pleural effusions are most common in this type of patient. Because complete relaxation is practically impossible to attain, these thyroid-type tuberculous patients go from bad to worse and seldom last more than a year or two after cavitation begins. Laboratory reports of their urine show impairment of kidney function, specifically in the excretion of carbonates, phosphates or sulphates. Blood count shows advanced secondary anemia and paucity of white cells. The sedimentation is markedly subnormal.

If the thyroid-type tuberculous patient is the bane of the nurses' life, the *adrenal type* of sufferer is the ward's favorite tonic—cheerful, easygoing, convivial. He never worries, usually laughs at new complications of his disease and is the most patient soul in the hospital. It is relatively easy to make him gain weight, for the day's high points are the sounds of the food cart in the hall. His digestion is good and he is seldom constipated. It is possible for him to stand more treatments, operations and even more lung hemorrhages than any other type of patient. His glandular equation would approximately be: Pituitary 50; Thyroid 25; Adrenals 100. He is the patient most often discharged as arrested or cured. All the treatment necessary for his recovery is supplied by bed rest and fresh air. Urine examination reveals normal kidney function. His blood count and sedimentation time are within normal limits.

And now we come to the patient who presents the greatest problem of all—the *pituitary type*. With a glandular equation of approximately Pituitary 100, Thyroid 75, Adrenals 25, he becomes a real problem. Depleted adrenals give him his characteristic weakness, cyanosis, cold hands and feet, poor digestion and constipation. His overstimulated pituitary enhances brain activity and makes it more difficult for him to forget his occupation, especially if it is mental in nature. He thinks and wonders and speculates all day long and can ask the attending physician more questions than three ordinary minds could explain. Besides being extremely unhappy in sanitarium surroundings, his inexhaustible sex energy, always seeking natural outlet, constitutes an added drain on his weak adrenals; any female, be she ward maid, nurse or scrub woman, is the target for his lascivious barrage. Another serious complication is his inordinate craving for coffee, alcohol or narcotics. Very few patients of this type make a recovery. Thin, tall, gaunt, nose and lips cyanotic or blue, they hobble about with cane or crutches, always darkly brooding.

The younger they are when cavitation begins, the shorter the duration of the disease and the quicker the end. It is not unusual for their sexual irritation to assert itself and find consummation either naturally or manually up to the very day of their deaths. Many of the great artists who died of tuberculosis belonged to this group. Here again is indication that the sex center lies in the pituitary gland and is only reinforced by the thyroid and adrenals.

Can you see yourself, wholly or in part, in these three gland types? The experienced eye of the physician can generally see much more of your emotional state than you can and he can direct treatment to your endocrine system, which is responsive to emotional states.

So you see that a knowledge of gland characteristics affords not only an interesting method of classifying types of patients, but, equally important, also helps the doctor to understand psychic behavior and temperament; to break down difficult mental barriers and to fathom, as Dr. S. Wier Mitchell was fond of saying, "the very soul of the patient."

It follows, then, that the more complete the understanding between doctor and patient, the greater the possibility for perfect co-operation, upon which depends the greatest likelihood of a cure.

PART II

WHEN THE MAGNIFICENT HUMAN BODY BREAKS DOWN

9

When Disease Strikes Children

Every physician is aware of the urgent queries crowding the minds of his puzzled patients. He would like to be able to answer all the questions relating to the particular disease of each of them, but time does not permit.

Because of this, I have attempted, in the following chapters, to explain something of the nature and causes of various diseases and offer guidance toward their alleviation or cure through proper management and diet. It is my belief that when the magnificent human body breaks down, it can be made whole again by correct diet. Though my own knowledge of these perplexing problems of disease and diet has been gained through many, many years of study and experience, it must be borne in mind that I can offer here only a rudimentary understanding of many complex diseases, each of which covers many thick medical volumes.

"Doctor, is my baby all right?" is the first question of almost every woman when her child is born. I myself have heard the question thousands of times. If every mother's greatest wish is to have a truly healthy baby, why (in most cases) does she take such poor care of herself before the baby is born? And why does she feed her child from infancy to adulthood so improperly that illness inevitably results?

This century has been called "The Century of the Child" because of the tremendous interest in the physical and psychological growth of children. But as we look around us, where are these radiantly healthy children? Certainly their parents are anxious to rear healthy youngsters. Some eight thousand books on child care have been published in the last twenty-five years. Why then are the offices of the country's thousands of pediatricians and general practitioners filled with runny-nosed, tired, allergic, feverish, run-down, anemic, bespectacled, acne-ridden, too thin or obese children?

The answer is simple:

(1) The mother's body was no fit environment for the child because her system was filled with waste products from improper food, drug residues, coffee acids, the poisons of cigarettes and alcohol.

(2) The growing child is improperly fed, spends too much time watching television, is driven everywhere instead of walking and devotes too little time to exercising in fresh air.

Can you blame me if I am filled with righteous indignation when I *know* that a healthy, happy baby is a sight to gladden the eye and cheer the heart of the onlooker at the nursery window in the hospital? I *know*, too, how lovely a sparkling, healthy new mother can be. I hope I won't be considered too boastful when I say that you can pick my patients out on the maternity wards—they're pink and pretty and in excellent spirits. No physician objects to being complimented by other physicians and by nurses. My patients do not have "caked breasts," fever, milk-leg, breast complications or uterine involution. With rare exceptions, pregnancies that I have attended through the whole nine months have had no problems. My patients have eaten properly during their pregnancies, remained at the proper weight, cleansed their systems of toxemia in order to give their babies a healthful environment; their labors, for the most part, were easy and without incident. Their children consequently grow up far healthier than the average.

The health of the "average" child is pretty low. And when you consider that almost five million children are born in the United States each "population-exploded" year, this is a grim fact. It has been estimated that it costs upward of $20,000 to raise a child to maturity. Statistics show, for instance, that 52 percent of our young men between 1948 and 1952 were rejected for military service on physical and mental grounds. Is this because, as children, their parents were too poor to provide healthful food? No, for many of the "overprivileged" children among them gorged themselves on chemical-ridden candy, cookies, ice cream, sweetened cola drinks, pancakes bathed in white-sugar syrups, popcorn and chocolate milk instead of obtaining the proper essential proteins, carbohydrates, fats and vitamins.

The tender years of childhood should be the healthiest of all. It is during those early years that the endocrine glands and liver are in their best functional capacity, giving the healthy child his natural state of exuberance, inexhaustible energy and faultless elimination. His bones should be strong as green oak, his teeth as indestructible as ivory, his hair thick, luxurious and lustrous.

Instead, the average baby comes into the world with his body full of toxins from the mother's blood and an intestine full of meconium (black oxidized bile). He is, in fact, so toxic that even with the best care it usually takes three years to eliminate his inherited birth poisons.

Nature tries to cleanse the mother's blood by sidetracking its impurities into the body of the infant. The first-born child is the most toxic and usually the most difficult to feed and rear. In the old days, when large families were popular or unavoidable, the fifth, sixth or seventh child often bloomed with unusual physical and mental vigor; when the mother gave birth to the tenth or twelfth, the children showed signs of the mother's glandular deterioration and exhaustion.

The first child usually presents many problems to the mother and her doctor. For example, a toxic excess of protein acids in the child will result, according to their concentration, in severe, then milder, then simple, or chronic manifestations of protein acid toxemia. The result of such conditions, I believe, can be early cancer (rare) or, later, leukemia (blood cancer) or other forms of slower-growing malignancies. Lesser concentrations can result in such diseases as rheumatism with or without valvular complications, polio, diphtheria, skin diseases or tonsillitis. This theory of the problems of the firstborn is one based on my personal research. A few other authorities in dietary medicine agree with me.

If the mother is tuberculous, the characteristic liver defect may be inherited and the child carried away with an early miliary tuberculosis. If starch indigestion is the source of the toxemia, the child will have the usual mucous diseases, from a mild respiratory rattling during babyhood to the chronic running nose of childhood, in which state the inflamed mucous membranes are a hotbed for every germ of infectious or contagious disease that comes along. When this type of child goes to kindergarten, it begins a gamut of infections and fevers and pneumonias that frightens the mother. If toxic fatty acids predominate as the source of toxemia, acne, styes, boils and carbuncles are the rule.

The general manifestations of disease in childhood are malaise, fatigue, mucus discharge from respiratory passages, skin rashes, nausea, vomiting and fever (fever may in some cases be absent). These common symptoms always indicate that (1) the blood is charged with poison; (2) the liver is unable to oxidize and neutralize it completely; (3) the offending acid is seeking elimination vicariously through skin and mucous membranes.

Germs, viruses and other microörganisms are usually present, but merely as scavengers that feed on toxic wastes. While we must thank Louis Pasteur for annihilating the belief that disease was caused by demons and devils, substituting in its place the germ theory, we must not forget that Beauchamp, who was a contemporary of Pasteur, strongly maintained that the chemical background on which the germ fed was of *equal importance*. Man had to choose between the two causes of disease: either the toxic background, due to faulty living and eating habits, was responsible for disease; or a mysterious microörganism, hiding in dark corners, pounced upon the innocent and unsuspecting victim. The cure, according to this latter theory, depended upon the destruction of these microbes.

We must remember, in discussing germs and disease, that what the germ *eats* is just as important as the germ itself. Without necessary food, the germ cannot live and thrive—and destroy. This explanation of disease serves to illustrate the importance of toxic waste products, inherited and acquired, and their relation to the diseases of childhood.

MEASLES

The measles germ, now thought to be a virus, thrives on a mucus exudate found in the upper respiratory tract. It may assume epidemic proportions, depending upon the concentration of the toxic waste products being eliminated vicariously through the mucous membranes. Symptoms in the following order appear: First, malaise and fatigue, which indicate liver toxemia; then fever, which is the result of the liver's attempt to oxidize the poison. Next, there are symptoms of a violent cold, with nasal discharges and cough; finally, the skin rash appears. After the liver has failed to oxidize all of the toxins, the thyroid gland helps as a third line of defense, eliminating the poisons through the inside skin or mucous membrane as an irritating catarrhal exudate, and through the outside skin as a rash. If the mucous membrane of the eye (conjuctiva) is involved, redness and photophobia result.

Sick children seldom eat (sick animals also refuse food), but occasionally they do or are forced to. Complications often follow. *Please do not force food on a sick child.*

How to treat measles? It is best treated as a severe cold. Baths or sponges help to reduce fever by enhancing elimination through the skin. Enemas carry away catarrhal bowel excretions as well as toxic bile eliminated by the liver, and should be given once or twice daily during the course of the disease. Nothing at all should be given by mouth except cracked ice, if desired. Later, diluted fruit juices for thirst as long as fever is present. Twenty-four hours after restoration of normal temperature, cooked non-starchy vegetables and cooked and raw fruit may be added. Two or three days later, when the rash has entirely disappeared, normal diet may be resumed.

It is dangerous to give aspirin or similar anti-pyretic drugs, since they only paralyze the nerve endings, offer a false sense of security

and increase the liver toxemia. Other drugs, used to suppress the
catarrh or the skin rash, tend to drive the toxins inward and damage internal organs. As the child needs physical rest, bed rest, so
do his mucous membranes, skin, liver and kidneys need chemical
rest, and this is effected *only through fasting*.

It is my belief that measles heads the list of the diseases of childhood which are the result of starch and sugar toxemia. Whooping
cough, croup, pneumonia, meningitis, influenza, sinusitis accompanied by a heavy nasal discharge, pink eye, bronchitis and asthma
are members of the same group. The natural antidote consists of
diluted fruit juices, such as apple, orange, grapefruit, pineapple,
papaya and guava.

A large group of childhood diseases originate, I feel, from protein acids, hereditary or aquired. These acids are not eliminated via
the mucous membranes, but through the lymphatic system, which
touches the mucous membranes in the nose and throat, such as
tonsils and small island patches of lymphatic tissue. Diseases of
the tonsils, pharynx, adenoids, middle ear and mastoid, and diphtheria, polio, typhoid, rheumatism and rheumatic heart disease all
come from protein acid intoxication: While milk is the best protein for the growing child, please remember that when, besides being pasteurized, it is boiled, dried and powdered, frozen as ice cream
or soured, fortified with synthetic vitamins, or mixed with chocolate
syrup, *it is unfit for food*. I cannot stress this too strongly. All of
these milk products putrefy in the child's intestine and give rise to
harmful protein acids.

TONSILLITIS

The most common site of vicarious elimination is the tonsil—a
lymph gland located on the surface of the mucous membrane of
the throat—which represents the terminal point of a chain of
similar, deeper lymph glands running from the intestinal region
upward in branching chains (in the neck as the cervical chains).

When toxic protein acids are shunted to the surface, their irritation may be so violent as to cause an acute burn (inflammation) of the tonsillar tissues, which is called tonsillitis. Sometimes the poison does not reach the tonsil but is blocked by one or more cervical lymph glands, which swell and cause painful "kernels" in the neck.

The superficial and accessible location of the tonsils make them an easy target for the surgeon, and many millions have been removed. The improvement that follows is largely the result of the self-imposed *fast* which attends the painful after-effects of the operation. The throat is too inflamed and sore to make swallowing possible. Later, the body, being devoid of these two most valuable portals of exit, seeks other areas where lymphatic (tonsillar) tissue touches mucous membranes. Lymphatic islands in the nose, throat, sinuses, stomach, bowel and appendix all attempt to carry on for the sacrificed tonsil, and a host of new diseases may follow, appendicitis heading the list.

POLIO

Polio, although really a comparatively rare disease, with mild symptoms such as fever, head cold and stiff neck, causes a pitiful muscular paralysis in about 2 percent of those afflicted. Although I believe that any toxic protein acid could cause the disease (said to be the result of a virus feeding upon waste eliminated through the lymphatic channels of the upper respiratory tract), I also believe that the most common source of the particular acid the polio virus seems to prefer comes from the putrefaction of ice cream in the bowels. Polio strikes most viciously at children who eat large quantities of ice cream. One indication of this is that the majority of cases occur during the peak of the summer ice-cream season. Middle-ear and mastoid disease, on the other hand, I believe, are most frequently the result of the child's eating eggs or foods containing eggs.

RHEUMATISM

One of the most unnecessary and tragic blights of childhood, rheumatism, comes mainly from the ingestion of meats and meat soups. Meat, although stimulating, is one of the most dangerous foods for the child. Its acids are vicariously sidetracked into the joint spaces, and if the blood becomes too concentrated, the heart valves (which are extremely sensitive to acids in the blood) can be damaged. Rheumatic heart or endocarditis is frequently the result of too much meat in the child's diet.

The natural antidotes for the protein acid diseases are the juices (raw or cooked) of vegetables, preferably non-starchy and well diluted. For the acute attack, a fast on diluted vegetable juice or soup is preferable but the canned product should never be used. Nor should salt, monosodium glutamate, meat or meat bone be added to soups for children suffering from rheumatism. For chronic intoxications, such as enlarged cervical lymph glands, simply eliminate all protein in the child's diet, using fruits, vegetables, starches and butter (a fat which, although a milk product, is unharmed by the pasteurization temperature), until the swelling has disappeared. Although protein, especially the right kind, is vitally needed for the growing child, it is often given to excess or in a devitalized state. Remember that the child grows less rapidly than a calf, so that it does not need as much milk as a calf. *Remember, too, that milk is a food, not a drink.*

Excessive ingestion of fat may also be harmful to the child. What is called a "fat" injury to the liver can be hereditary or can be acquired after birth. Because of disturbance to the liver cells, dietary fat, mostly cream in the case of the young child, is not completely oxidized and circulates in the blood as a toxic fat. This is eliminated either through the hair fat glands (one at the base of each hair to oil it) or through the sebaceous glands (which naturally oil the skin). *Seborrhea capitus,* commonly known as "cradle cap," is an example of the first; acne, pimples, small pustules (commonly seen on the chest, abdomen, genitals and anus of the infant), or styes, boils and abscesses (when eliminated through the sebaceous glands) may develop. If the fat in the bone marrow is involved, the result would be osteomyelitis (abscesses in the bone marrow). The cure depends upon proper drainage of the pus and withdrawal of all fat from the diet, especially the fat in all forms of shortening.

CHICKEN POX

The most common acute disease of childhood which results from a fat toxemia is chicken pox, a highly contagious disease—hardly any children escape it. I believe it to be due to the elimination of toxic fat or fatty acids through the hair fat glands, which is the natural food of a virus. The chemical burn from the excretory products of this microörganism causes the characteristic blister of this disease. Smallpox and diphtheria, now both very rare, have long since been cleaned up by the sanitary engineers.

The medical treatment of childhood diseases can be classified under two headings: anti-pyretic and stimulant. In treatment by anti-pyretics, aspirin tops the list of favorites. Aspirin is related to carbolic acid. Over a hundred years ago, a drop of carbolic acid on a lump of sugar was taken for relief of pain, headache or fever.

Aspirin is the German chemists' highest synthetic realization. It is a phenol (carbolic acid) derivative, with all the chemical qualities of phenol but without the deadly effect of carbolic acid. If the urine is tested after taking aspirin, a positive test for phenol is present. Aspirin, like phenol, deadens the nerve endings, thereby masking pain. Headache, fatigue or indisposition diminish. Aspirin also diminishes the fever by partially blocking the thyroid and the adrenal glands. But the phenol derivatives interfere with the proper function of the liver and damage liver cells. The use of aspirin, then, is an attempt to drive out one devil (disease toxins) by admitting another devil!

Fever in a child is a frightening symptom to the mother. Just what is the function of fever? Is it a harmful process, something to suppress and worry about? Or is it the body's attempt to burn up a poison, thereby helping to dispose of it more quickly?

In the diseases of childhood, fever begins in the liver. In a very strong, robust child, with properly functioning endocrine glands, the toxin is often completely consumed in the liver. The child does not feel sick or have pain; it just has a fever and if the liver area is carefully palpated, it can be noted that there is an elevation of temperature over that organ. In fact, if the temperature under the tongue is 105 degrees, the internal temperature of the liver may be as high as 110 degrees. But if the liver is unable to oxidize completely the poisons of disease so that some leak through into the blood stream, then, under the action of the endocrine glands, the poisons seek vicarious outlets via the mucous membranes. This may be through the upper respiratory tract, in the form of flu, sinusitis, pharyngitis, tonsillitis and possibly even pneumonia, which is a complicated kind of bronchitis. All through this process, the whole power of the liver is diverted into neutralizing the toxic wastes of disease, as evidenced by the fever.

The liver is much too busy to be bothered with the task of the digestion of food. Great strain can be taken off that organ if *no food* is given. While the fire is burning, nature does not want food. That is why animals and many children refuse food when disease is present. Not only does fasting lower the temperature, relieve the distress and facilitate elimination, but it also lessens the strain on the liver and prevents serious complications, such as middle-ear disease, mastoiditis and meningitis.

My own observations over half a century of active practice have taught me that the fast (on cracked ice, diluted fruit or vegetable juices) should be continued for twenty-four hours after the temperature has returned to normal.

A good rule to remember is that the bowel can be cleared of toxins (by physic or enemas) in *twenty-four hours;* the blood in *three days;* the liver in *five days, providing no food is eaten.*

It appears then, that fever, dreaded because misunderstood, is really nature's attempt to help. It never does harm; never is attended with serious aftereffects and never should be suppressed with drugs or fed with food. I have seen many a case of flu pushed into a pneumonia because some anxious grandmother insisted upon something "to give the child strength," such as chicken broth or a thin starchy gruel, both liquids, of course, but protein and starch—just what the liver cannot handle at this point.

The second classification of treatment of childhood diseases comes under the heading of stimulants—chemical whips which accelerate the action of the thyroid and adrenal glands. In earlier days Abraham Jacobi, considered the father of pediatrics, used as much as a pint of whiskey a day for a child suffering from an attack of pneumonia. It was his chief stimulating drug. Today the sulfas, antibiotics and steroid drugs are the popular glandular whips. And though it may be hard to believe, their aftereffects are distinctly more harmful than Jacobi's alcohol, which the body was able to burn and eliminate quickly. Stimulating an exhausted body by means of drugs is just as nonsensical as whipping a tired horse to make it work. It is far safer to rest the animal, put it in pasture (where it will feed on clean, high-vitamin food) and give it a chance to build up its strength.

There are no miracles, no short cuts, in medicine. Nature does her work in a slow, methodical way, as a tree grows. Man's attempt to hurry the process too often ends in disaster.

FEEDING THE BABY

Of all the perplexing problems in infant feeding, indigestion presents the most worrisome one. The chief cause of this indigestion is toxic bile, which is usually acid but should be alkaline. Symptoms such as gas, colic, pains, nervousness and insomnia are common. It is important for the mother to understand the source and cause of this toxic bile (usually green instead of the normal golden yellow) and thereby better understand her baby's ailments.

The blood that is used for the nourishment and development of the unborn baby is kept pure by the action of three filters: the first is the mother's liver, the second is the afterbirth, which stands as a second line of defense against toxic material circulating toward the infant; the third is the infant's own liver, through which the blood of the umbilical cord circulates *before* it enters the general circulation of the baby's body.

The toxic bile which remains in the baby's liver is gradually eliminated during the first three years of the infant's life. At certain intervals this toxic green-colored bile is thrown into the baby's bowel for elimination. When this happens all the disagreeable symptoms of infant indigestion follow. Milk is transformed into rubbery curds which are identified as hard bean-sized masses in the stool. Starches and sugars ferment, giving rise to gas and colic and strong intestinal pain of the knife-cutting variety. Even the best human milk is improperly digested. *The fault lies in the chemistry of the baby's liver and not in the nourishment given.* Too often attention is focused upon the baby's diet instead of the baby's chemistry. As a result we have a most fantastic array of preparations that pass as nourishment for the ailing infant. Usually one after another is tried on the baby and in the course of time, provided it does not die from their effect, it is able to eliminate enough of the toxic green bile to be able to digest part of these commerically prepared and synthetic foods. Hence the last one tried gets the credit for curing the infant.

There is only one natural food for the baby: *milk.* It should be pure, fresh, preferably from nipple to mouth, and unadulterated. Mother's milk is always best, providing the mother is not too toxic. Goat's milk is next best and then cow's milk. Goat's or cow's milk should be diluted and sweetened to conform as nearly as possible to the composition of mother's milk. Milk that has stood for twenty-four hours, even though refrigerated, loses many of its valuable properties. The more it is heated and treated, the less nourishing it is as a food. The natural vitamins can never be replaced by synthetic ones. Pasteurization, though detrimental, is not entirely harmful, because some of the good qualities of the milk remain unchanged. The necessity for pasteurization is the penalty of city life and mass civilization. Very little or no nourishment is left in boiled or superheated, canned or dried milk or milk powder.

As the child grows and gains strength it will have more energy to be used for the elimination of toxins. These toxins are thrown out by the child's liver, via the bile, which is the normal excretory product of the liver. Normal bile is compatible with almost any kind of food that happens to be in the intestine; abnormal or toxic bile has an irritating effect upon the delicate intestinal lining. As toxic bile stops normal digestion of proteins, sugars, starches and fats, all the distressing symptoms of intestinal indigestion follow, the most marked being gas, colic, pain, constipation or diarrhea, nervous instability and a general restlessness.

During the acute phases of the bile crisis practically no digestion is possible, therefore it is best to limit the diet to distilled water or greatly diluted fruit juices or vegetable soup made of the juice of cooked alkaline vegetables, with no meat broth. It may be necessary to continue this program from one to three days. When the crisis has subsided, the baby should be fed. It is best to begin with a formula of dilute raw cow's milk, half milk and half water.

The minimum requirement of nourishment for the first six months of the infant's life is sixteen ounces of milk per twenty-four hours. For bottle-fed babies, the milk should be diluted with distilled water. The amount of dilution depends upon the baby's ability to handle it. When sweetening can be tolerated, brown or raw sugar or honey is preferable to the synthetic syrups, molasses, powdered lactose or commercial glucose. If sugars cause gas and colic, skin rashes, diarrhea, scorching of the skin around the anus and general restlessness, they should be eliminated from the baby's diet until the reaction of the bile becomes more normal, at which time the sweetening can be tolerated. Starches and fats are always poorly digested during the first year of life. After that, if there remains any degree of indigestion, they should not be given.

The proper dilution of the milk and the spacing of the feedings is an art that demands careful attention from an ever observant mother. A constant juggling of the proportions of milk and water may be necessary. The sole criterion is the reaction and behavior of the baby.

It will be heartening for the new mother to know that as the days and weeks roll by for the child with toxic bile, the attacks of indigestion lessen. Sugar and fruit juices, fruits and vegetables can now be tolerated and eventually digested with ease and comfort. But in any event it is dangerous to try to suppress the bile crisis with chemicals or drugs. Co-operation with nature will allow the baby's body to eliminate its inherited toxins. Temporary palliative treatment will plague the health of the child in later years and possibly deform its teeth and bones. Patience, loving care and a heroic determination that overcomes worry, loss of sleep and irregular meals eventually reward the mother with a healthy and beautiful child.

Emerson once said that the child who is able to walk is presumed to be well. In discussing the ills of children I have taken up a good deal of space to show you what "to be well" really means and the myriad of ills which can attack the below-par child. I know that if there were more radiantly healthy children I would see fewer sick adults in my office. For true health begins not in childhood—but in the mother's womb.

10

Cholesterol and the
Troubled Heart

One of the most fearsome and misunderstood words today is cholesterol. Possibly the least knowledgeable was the patient who declared vehemently: "I'm just not going to let one speck of that cholesterol creep into my blood! I don't know too much about it, but I do know it's poison. Is it true, Doctor, that it's a combination of that plant stuff chlorophyll and that medicine Geritol?"

More informed people are equally worried about cholesterol and its relationship to heart impairment, because they have read that while polio is a relatively minor disease in terms of numbers of humans afflicted, heart disease, according to statistics, kills more Americans than all other illnesses combined—thirteen hundred men and women every day, nearly one every minute, and brain strokes snuff out another five hundred lives daily.

Long before cholesterol became a household word, I had spent a good deal of time studying it and its relation to the troubled heart in order to determine if impure food made impure cholesterol. And I arrived, I believe, at a logical explanation of the cholesterol problem and a logical method of building a pure cholesterol in the body.

One of the most hotly debated questions in medicine today concerns cholesterol: Is it or is it not the villain in heart disease? What is at the root of the cholesterol-heart disease controversy—cholesterol in your food, in your blood, in your arteries?

To begin with, perfect health depends upon the condition of the arteries through which the blood circulates to reach every living cell of the body. This current of blood is unbelievably strong, rushing with the turbulence of the swiftest mountain stream. But while the banks of the mountain stream are altered by erosion, the body tissues are unaffected by the violent currents of blood. How is this possible? Protection is afforded by the lubrication of the lining of the arterial walls. Nature has perfected a frictionless substance which keeps the body from being washed away by its own blood currents. The key element of this most effective lubrication oil is a fat-like substance called cholesterol.

The word cholesterol is most complex, deriving from the Greek *chole* (bile) and *stereos* (solid) and from the Latin *olium* (oil). It is also a most complex hydrocarbon, yellowish-white in color and fatty to the touch, perfectly composed for the important part it has to play in maintaining smoothness for the circulation of the blood. Even if every trace of cholesterol is omitted from the diet, it continues to circulate in the blood, for the liver manufactures it.

During the development of the embryo, cholesterol is supplied by the mother's blood. After birth the child must manufacture its own. The oil needed for this, nature supplies in the most useful fat, cream, otherwise known as butterfat. One of the important functions of the liver is the synthesis of cholesterol from butterfat. Of course, other vegetable and animal fats can be used, but during the stage of the child's early development, butterfat is supplied by the mother's milk.

The cholesterol, built up by the liver cells from simple fats, circulates in the blood in just the proper concentration to be utilized by the cells which line the artery walls, and is held there as the perfect lubricant. As these cells wear out, they are cast off, together with their cholesterol, and excreted by the body, while new cells grow and absorb new cholesterol from the blood. Thus, there occurs a continuous in-and-out flow of cholesterol, which, as long as the body is in perfect health, is maintained at a specific level.

When the physiological level of the cholesterol is disturbed by a more rapid breaking-down than building-up process, the overall cholesterol concentration in the blood is increased and there occurs a state of *hypercholestremia, i.e.*, too much cholesterol in the blood. There are simple laboratory tests by which the amount of circulating cholesterol can be determined.

The only condition that can cause a more rapid breaking-down than building-up of cholesterol is a diseased state of the artery walls. *Overeating of fats and oils, as long as they are in their natural state, cannot cause arterial disease.* The body merely stores the excess as fat.

It is only when *unnatural* fats, or *natural fats which have been altered by being overheated,* are consumed as food, that the trouble arises. Especially is the composition of the fat altered when it is heated with starch (for example, French-fried potatoes). I have found that it is impossible for the liver to synthesize a perfect cholesterol from a fat that has been heated with starch. The resulting cholesterol is used by the body for arterial lining, but being an unnatural or altered cholesterol, it fails to wear well, soon breaks down and is corroded, resulting in various forms of arterial disease and degeneration—arteriosclerosis (commonly called hardening or narrowing of the artery walls, which causes them to lose their elasticity); atherosclerosis (fatty deposits on the arterial walls, which may impede or even block the blood flow); coronary thrombosis (blood clotting in the arteries, which blocks the blood supply to the heart); and aneurism (ruptured tumor in artery wall). In these states the concentration of cholesterol in the blood is much higher than the normal level. The increased level can be detected early by the alert physician as a danger signal which will lead him to make a study of the patient's fat metabolism.

The idea that a high-fat diet is necessarily harmful to the arteries—although currently immensely popular with physicians—is contradicted by a careful study of the diet of Eskimos. These people, before their primitive diet was contaminated by the refined foods of civilization, were among the strongest and healthiest on earth. They lived entirely on meat, fish, fowl *and* a great deal of fat. Like the seal and the walrus, they needed a thick layer of body fat to serve as an insulation against the freezing weather. And, again like the seal and the walrus, they easily oxidized their fat which served as a source of heat and energy.

It is true that they matured and aged early, but that was not because of a faulty diet. Rather, the rigorous ordeal of weather and the long Arctic night was the cause. Their bones were stronger than those of any other race of man, their strength was prodigious and their health phenomenal. Although on a high-fat diet, and a so-called "saturated" fat intake at that, their blood cholesterol was normal and their arteries perfect. (Saturation is explained later in this chapter.) Once when the explorer Vilhjalmur Stefansson was living with the Eskimos, enjoying superb health on their native diet, he decided to experiment by abstaining from fat, so he selected the leanest meat and fish procurable. In a few weeks he grew violently weak and ill. His Eskimo friends begged him to include large quantities of fat in his diet or he would die. Stefansson followed their advice and made a quick recovery.

It is only natural for physicians and scientific experts on body metabolism to assume that a high-fat diet parallels increased blood cholesterol. The factor which seems to have been overlooked (and one which I originally formulated) is that *normal dietary fats are altered not only by overheating, but by being heated in contact with other substances that make them unfit for the manufacture of the perfect arterial lining.*

As civilized man's diet gradually became more unnatural he began to suffer not only from disturbances of fat metabolism but also from carbohydrate and protein indigestion, resulting in a general toxemia of the blood. I believe that to be the primary cause of many, perhaps of all, diseases. The finding of a high blood cholesterol, therefore, indicates the presence of a disturbance in fat metabolism as well as in the metabolism of carbohydrates and proteins. Thus, it harbors a high degree of body toxemia.

There is much fearful discussion these days over "saturated" and "unsaturated" fats and their harmfulness or usefulness in the diet. Naturally, people are deeply interested in cholesterol's role in heart and artery disease, but many are misinformed.

The easiest way to understand the difference between a "saturated" and "unsaturated" fat can be demonstrated by this example:

Let us visualize two men: one, a normal person with two arms and hands, capable of holding objects; the other fashioned like a Hindu god with many waving arms and hands. When the normal man holds, let us say, two apples, his hands are full. When the Hindu god holds two apples, his hands are not full, for he has many other hands with which to grasp apples. The two-handed man is saturated, the other unsaturated (with apples). Chemistry would say that the normal man has two open *bonds* that are saturated. The Hindu god would have many bonds, not saturated, but open and able to grasp and hold other chemical substances. In chemical laboratory parlance, it would be said that the many-handed man has a higher *valence* than the two-handed man.

Valences of substances are often tested in the laboratory. Because the element iodine easily attaches itself to open bonds, it is used to determine the saturation point of open-bonded compounds. Free iodine is mixed with a substance, and then is searched for. If the open bonds of the substance have grasped the iodine, there remains no more free iodine and the amount grasped is called the "iodine value" of the formerly unsaturated substance. When a substance becomes "saturated," its chemical reactions are altered; an irritating toxin can become a benign compound. The action of many of the useful drugs depends upon the same principle; for instance, it is possible to "digitalize" a body poison by giving a patient digitalis, and to "iodize" a poison by giving potassium iodide, an ancient specific for toxemia. The current vogue is to neutralize with unsaturated fats, which are really therapeutic buffers.

As a neutralizing agent, or buffer, unsaturated hydrocarbons are of value in treating toxic conditions of the body. But, in some cases, instead of leaving unsaturated cooking oils and margarine in their natural states, commercialism has again stepped in, altered their melting points to make them resemble butter or other natural shortenings, "fortified" them with synthetic "vitamins," added monosodium glutamate or glutamic acid, aniline-dye coloring matter, salt and traces of butter or cream for special flavor. Actually, all of these additives tend to saturate the hydrocarbons so that the final product, pleasing to the taste and gratifying to the mind of the consumer, is little more than glorified grease!

What fats, then, are healthful for the body?

The answer can only be—the *natural, unadulterated* fats. Animal fats, which include meat fats, organ fats, marrow fats and brain fats; vegetable fats, such as the fat in beans, seeds, nuts, avocados, bananas and other tropical fruits including papayas, mangoes, sapotas and coconuts. As far as their usefulness to the body is concerned, it makes little difference whether they are *saturated* or *unsaturated*, provided the liver is healthy enough to synthesize them for the blood.

But fats, saturated or unsaturated, do their greatest harm to the body when they are used as shortening or cooking oil, that is, when they are heated with other foods, especially the starches. Fried bread or potatoes, doughnuts, hot cakes, pie crust, cakes and pastries—all offer *altered* cholesterol. And when you eat these highly regarded confections, the result is imperfect artery lining, erosion of the arteries, atherosclerosis. The greatest offenders are doughnuts and potato chips, with popcorn a close third (before popcorn will "pop," it must be heated in cooking oil).

Many a bustling young executive between the age of thirty and forty-five has fallen victim of a stroke or a coronary. Because he felt he was too rushed to eat a proper meal, he had developed the habit of eating doughnuts and coffee several times a day. Munching on potato chips or popcorn while watching TV or reading is a widespread and dangerous habit. And the surest way to render cooked string beans or other vegetables indigestible is to saturate or "season" them with bacon grease.

One of the most pitiful examples of chronic altered cholesterol poisoning is seen in a condition called Buerger's disease, characterized by a gangrenous rotting of the arteries, most often seen in the extremities. It is generally believed now that Buerger's disease is caused by cigarette smoking. The heat of the burning tobacco and paper literally "fries" the oils and tars of the tobacco with the carbohydrate of the leaf and paper, resulting in a poisonously altered fat or oil. Although, happily, advanced cases of Buerger's disease are rare, there are thousands of victims suffering from mild intoxication, cold hands and feet, numbness and tingling fingers that turn blue or white, deformities of the nails and teeth. Most of these sufferers, post mortem, show obliterated coronary arteries.

At the present time, diseases of the heart, which include diseases of the blood vessels, are the greatest killers of the human race, especially in civilized countries. A more careful selection and use of dietary fats would lessen the number of these victims. Although the human body is a marvelous machine, it cannot build sound, healthy tissues from foods that have been grossly adulterated for commercial purposes.

The heart is the center of the body's transportation system. It is a muscle, the most important one in the body because it pumps blood to all the other muscles and tissues. Yet it must have blood for its own use, if it is to do its work. If the blood supply is cut off for only a few minutes, the heart ceases to carry out its work.

Since the leading killers in our country today are diseases which impair the heart, there is, naturally, a tremendous interest in this miraculous little muscle. Shaped like a fist, it begins to beat before birth, and appears to work constantly, night and day thereafter. But physiologists tell us that during the functioning of an organ, many of its cells are in the resting phase, a fact that has been amply demonstrated in the laboratory in connection with liver and kidney function. This is especially true of the heart, which, although constantly beating, not only rests between contractions but seldom calls for the united action of all of its muscle cells except in times of emergency.

The untiring muscular pump is a wonderfully efficient and tough organ; it can pump blood either at a high or low efficiency level, as occasion demands. This ability to respond to demand is the result first of the rate of the beat and second of the force of the beat. Under extreme duress the heart is capable of tremendous increase in efficiency; when necessary a compensatory stretching and enlargement occurs, until the organ increases to half again its normal size. When this happens, all of its muscle cells work at an optimum rate. The characteristic tortuosity of the coronary vessels make this stretching possible. Fortunately, the valves and *chorda tendinae* (small fibrous cords that support the valves) are able to endure this tremendous strain; in a few days after the crisis has passed, the heart regains its normal size and equilibrium.

Naturally, there is a physiological limit to this response. In studies of the action of the hearts of normal animals under such strain as is involved in prolonged flight or a state of fright, no resulting damage to the animal's heart has ever been observed which is in any way comparable to the human "heart attack." If, however, the animal is taken out of its environment, he becomes much more susceptible to disease.

Man, too, has been removed from his original environment. He must breathe the impure air of cities; he is subjected to emotional and physical stress and strain; his eardrums are assailed with irritating and sometimes unbearable noises with consequent disturbed rest at night; he suffers from unnatural tensions, anxieties and intense eyestrain from fatigue, such as is occasioned by improper lighting of streets and roads; he must drink chemicalized water and eat synthetic food.

Under such circumstances, instead of a physiological man, we have a *pathological* man, whose heart becomes as pathological as he and as incapable of enduring stress and strain. Inevitably, then, the heart muscle loses its tone; the valves and *chordae* their elasticity; the vessels harden, the timing mechanism gets out of gear; the walls dilate until finally there is a fuel pump which cannot stand any kind of strain. A whole new pump or many new parts are necessary to restore the efficiency of a worn-out heart, for the heart is an engine, in many respects quite similar to a gasoline engine.

One comparison concerns the fuel. The gasoline makes power possible by oxidation. The gasoline is to the engine what the adrenal principle is to the heart, since the adrenal principle makes oxidation possible in the heart muscle. To regulate the gasoline motor, a carburetor is needed which prepares the fuel, turning it into a mixture the motor can utilize. The corresponding human carburetor is the thyroid gland. But the gas engine must be operated by a driver in order to perform properly. The counterpart of the driver is the pituitary gland. The ciliated nerve cells of this gland are bathed in the blood which circulates through its intermediary portion. The cells detect toxic substances, and through direct sympathetic nerve impulses regulate the body's defense mechanism. But here again nature shows her superiority over the engine of man's creation. The gas engine can develop more power only by increasing its speed; the heart is able not only to increase its speed but also its size, growing from a small engine to a large one, and later resuming its original size.

When a gasoline motor is improperly lubricated or the fuel is of poor grade or badly mixed, there can be corrosion, missing spark plugs, valve leaks and loss of power. But we take precious care of our automobiles while we subject our hearts to a series of insults that may, too often and too soon, cause its destruction. Every day, we read in the papers of sudden deaths and say, "Ah, another heart attack!" We are led to believe that "heart attacks," because they are common, are more or less necessary, perhaps even a polite and civilized way for nine hundred thousand Americans to die every year.

It stands to reason that the heart gradually becomes pathological when too many of the physiological rules of life have been broken. The degree of damage to the heart structure depends upon changes in the chemistry of the blood and responses to sudden adrenal hyperactivity caused by states of toxemia. Many of the so-called "pseudo anginas," as well as serious attacks of angina pectoris (constricting paroxysms of chest pain caused by insufficiency of blood), can be relieved by diluting the body fluids with water containing mild alkalis given by mouth or by rectum. This would indicate that the lining membrane of the heart valves is extremely sensitive to irritants or acids in the blood. As McKim Marriott says in *Recent Advances in Chemistry in Relation to Medical Practice:* ". . . The chemical difference between life and death is smaller than the difference between tap water and distilled water."

It is well understood how tenaciously the body maintains the neutrality of the blood and how other organs act as buffers and sidetracking stations of circulating toxins. And it is only when all these buffers are saturated that a minute, but often fatal, amount of toxins can circulate in the blood. Much damage can be done to the heart valves through chemical irritation, and the resulting inflammation often gives basal focus for the formation of germ colonies of the streptococcus group.

It was previously stated that the thyroid secretion controls the *rate* of the heartbeat and that states of paroxysmal tachycardia (increased rate of heartbeat, often to as high as 250 per minute) can result from an excess of the internal secretion of the thyroid gland in the blood. There are two general methods of combating this condition. When the adrenals are *hypo*active and the thyroid *hyper*active, as is frequently the case, any psychic or chemical stimulation of the adrenals may restore the balance between the two glands with resulting heart equilibrium. Or conversely, the action of the thyroid can be depressed by insulin, a drug with a powerful depressive action on the thyroid. Some years ago I was called to see a patient who had been in a state of paroxysmal tachycardia for more than sixty hours. He looked moribund. Fifteen units of insulin, repeated every fifteen minutes, restored him to normalcy in the course of three hours.

Another heart condition most alarming to the patient is that characterized by broken rhythm. This unrhythmic beating results from one of two causes. The first is an excessive spurt of internal secretion of the thyroid gland into the patient's blood, which creates a feeling of great and increasing apprehension. He is alarmed at the sudden jerking, the missing or the somersaulting of the heart together with a feeling that his brain is being violently disturbed. But clinical experience has taught us that this ailment seldom leads to a serious pathological state. The second cause is an irregularity resulting from a pathological degeneration of the nerve bundles in the heart muscle which leads to auricular fibrillation (or flutter) and heart block.

The most common of the heart disorders, the so-called "heart attack," nearly always follows a sudden increase of the adrenal principle in the circulation. The result is either an acute dilation or the rupture of a valve or muscular wall, the clot from the resultant hemorrhage doing much damage. There can also be a rupture of an inelastic coronary vessel. Any or all of these lesions may cause sudden death. The patients who recover do so because the damage has been from stretching only. Bed rest, light diet and oxygen often perform therapeutic miracles.

The sudden adrenal "bath" that so often overwhelms the patient in the form of a heart attack is a response of the defense mechanism against an acute toxemia resulting from chemical or nervous shock or both. I should like to repeat this statement because I believe so firmly that here is the primary cause of "heart attacks." The cause behind the cause, so to speak. *The sudden adrenal "bath" that so often overwhelms the patient in the form of a heart attack is the response of the defense mechanism against an acute toxemia resulting from chemical or nervous shock or both.*

If the liver and kidneys, which are the filters of the blood, are unable to cope with sudden intoxication, the result is that a great strain is put upon the heart because of the high toxemia of the blood. From internal congestion due to poisonous products in the blood the liver and kidneys slowly degenerate because this congestion interferes with their blood supply. Much can be done to relieve the strain on these filters. But many factors are involved. The chief circulation of blood through the liver is via the portal vein. When there is liver congestion, a back pressure of blood into the whole venous system occurs. With it comes a state of plethora, or increased vein pressure, which can easily be detected. Patients are always interested in tests to determine what is wrong with them. So here is a simple test for increased vein pressure, which is also the most valuable liver-function test and does not involve expensive laboratory procedure. Press down on the skin between the shoulder blades with back turned to a mirror or have someone do this. Remove the fingertips which have made the pressure. If a blanched, white area remains, it is an indication that increased vein pressure or plethora, exists. When the vein pressure is normal, no white area is noticeable. This same test may be made in other areas (the chest or legs), and will give the same result.

Although the individual may feel perfectly well, if this white area persists after the finger test, it means that there is trouble ahead, that the increased vein pressure is exerting harmful back-washes between venous and arterial blood. Increased auricular pressure in the right side of the heart where the vein blood enters can cause a sense of weight in the chest and if the left side of the heart, the ventricles, do not beat more forcibly, can cause the person to faint, which simply means that nature places him in the horizontal position until some balance between the venous and arterial pressure can be restored. This unnatural pressure between arterial and venous blood often causes back currents and whirlpools in the blood vessels of the ears, causing the common annoyance of ringing of the ears. In the semicircular canals of the labyrinth of the ears, this pressure may result in dizziness, nausea and even vomiting. In the eyes, conjunctival or even retinal hemorrhages may ensue. And so on elsewhere in the body, ad infinitum.

Veins are easily dilated. The results are venous or capillary varices or hemorrhages. In the heart, as a result of this stasis, the auricles have difficulty in emptying themselves. Conversely, the chief blood supply of the glomeruli of the kidneys is arterial. Glomeruli are tiny, globe-like filters in the kidneys, which can become inflamed and eventually may be destroyed, if the arterial blood is toxic. And if the glomeruli diminish in number because some of them have been destroyed, it means that the volume of blood circulating through the kidneys will also be diminished. To deliver a normal volume of filtered blood to the general circulation, blood must be pumped harder and faster in order to get the needed amount through the kidneys, and to do this the heart must necessarily increase the blood pressure; this naturally means emergency action on the part of the heart. A strong heart can elevate the blood pressure and stand the strain for years; weaker hearts dilate and eventually collapse as a result of this tremendous strain.

Particularly since ex-President Eisenhower's highly publicized coronary attack in 1955, it may perhaps be more distinguished to have a bad heart than a bad liver or more genteel to have a heart ailment than kidney trouble. But there is really very little difference, if one looks for initial causes. It must never be forgotten that the liver and kidneys are the filters of the body. *And it follows that if less therapeutic attention is paid to the pump and more is given to correcting the pathological conditions of the liver and kidneys, the pump will be less embarrassed.*

How can this be accomplished? The most reasonable procedure to insure normal and proper liver and kidney function is *not* to subject these organs to chemical strain. Albert Szent-Györgyi, noted Nobel Prize-winning biochemist, concluded that "The purity, the humidity and the temperature of the air, the quantity of noise and excitement, physical work, insulation, etc., are important. But certainly one of the most essential factors in our coordination with our surroundings is our food, for food is the form in which our surroundings penetrate into our body in rough, big quantities."

Proper choice and preparation of our food insures adequate vitamin intake, an important consideration if health is to be maintained. To put it in the simplest manner, everything revolves around the chemistry of digestion. A car will not run well on contaminated gasoline; nor will a body on poor food. The tremendous importance of a proper dietary regime is certainly the key to better general health as well as to *normal heart function.*

"One of the most important factors—if not the most important —in the incidence of coronary disease is the diet," declares cardiologist Myron Prinzmetal in his book *Heart Attack.* "It is palpably clear that we, as a rule, eat too much. Primitive people usually don't. They can't afford to stuff themselves. We seem to consider it a mark of affluence and luxury to eat big meals. When an American suddenly gets an increase in income, gets a raise in salary or puts over a big deal, he usually takes his family out to celebrate with what he calls a 'good' meal. The 'good' meal is always a high-caloric, fatty meal in which the family joins him in cramming more fuel into the system than the system can accommodate. Poor people in economically backward countries don't usually put over big deals; they don't take the family out for a big meal. They don't get coronaries."

Moderation should ever be the golden rule in the diet, especially for the heart patient. He should remember that a meal of many courses and heavy food throws a sudden load on the heart, which then is obliged to pump an extra supply of blood to digest it. Frequent small meals are better than overeating at any one meal or alternating between feast and famine. Sweet desserts and fat foods, including fatty meats and gravies, should give way to vegetable soup, lean meats, vegetables, salads and fruits.

In my opinion, at the present time, much of the diagnosis and treatment of heart ailments appears to be *an overemphasis in the wrong direction*. There has always been a compelling belief among the public that when disease occurs, the doctor must *do* something. And do it quickly. Primitive medicine men put on a great show, complete with colorful costumes, feathers and bizarre masks. Our present tendency sometimes suggests magic, with machines that spark or make sharp noises or emit disagreeable odors. Or we may puncture or shock the patient. And it must be admitted that many patients enjoy this complicated ritual. The prophetic voice of Sir William Osler, who observed: "It takes more courage to do nothing intelligently than to stuff the patient with drugs," has long been forgotten. There was also Sir James Mackenzie, who often wished that he had never invented the "polygraph" (great-grandfather of the electrocardiograph), because it disturbed him when he saw its findings so flagrantly misused in diagnosis.

Earlier Mackenzie had emphasized this idea when he said: "I want to impress upon you the fact that the means of investigation we possess in ourselves, without the use of mechanical devices, have not yet even begun to be employed." Internists of great hospitals have admitted that post-mortem findings very often differ greatly from the cardiograph diagnosis.

There have been a good many criticisms regarding the diagnosing of heart disease merely from electrocardiograms. Many physicians forget that "slurrings" and "notchings" occur routinely in those over thirty. Speaking of the cardiograph, the noted Dr. James C. Thomson of Edinburgh observed: "This highly complex and impressive piece of apparatus has a great suggestive value and produces interesting graphs, but it gives not the slightest inkling of some of the worst forms of disease, even at the terminal phases thereof. For example, edema, recognizable by the experienced clinician at first glance, may bring no indication whatever from these highly impressive instruments...."

Dr. Thomson continued: "To the cardiographic technician, the patient, as an individual, is rapidly lost sight of. Clinically, he ceases to exist once the practitioner's attention becomes fixed upon his instrument—a marvelous machine that makes soft purring sounds and produces complicated records. Meanwhile, to the fevered imagination of the frightened patient, each wriggling line is tangible proof of his direful condition—a detail not noticed by the practitioner, fascinated in his interpretation of the graphs. For him the patient has become a mere extension of the machine; an important adjunct for the production of even more perfect graphs. The cardiograph is, I believe, one of the factors responsible for much of the misunderstanding exhibited by specialists."

Many medical men agree with such opinions, particularly Dr. Francis F. Rosenbaum of Milwaukee, who said: "The electrocardiograph cannot tell the heart's whole story. If the graph shows a minor deviation from normal, the doctor usually mutters something about 'strain' and orders the patient to give up some of his favorite activities. This exaggerated caution causes many patients serious psychologic and economic suffering. False security, leading to overexertion, can be far more tragic. A man may have made a good recovery from one heart attack, so that his electrocardiogram looks almost normal. But at the very moment of the reading, a clot may be forming in a coronary artery which will kill him next day."

I do not recommend discarding the electrocardiograph. And neither does Dr. Rosenbaum. But he and many other physicians insist that its evidence be accepted as only *part* of the story—along with laboratory tests and thorough physical examination.

An illuminating case illustrating this point was that of a young California pro-football player who felt achy and feverish and complained of a slight chest pain. His doctor took an electrocardiogram, noted an unusual wave pattern in it and diagnosed a heart attack. For three years the patient remained incapacitated in the belief that he had suffered a heart attack, although he showed no symptoms whatever of heart disease. He became a semi-invalid and felt unable to do the lightest work. A complete re-examination uncovered no evidence of heart disease. His wave pattern was merely an unusual variation. Informed that he had no indication of heart trouble, the young man refused to believe it. A few sessions with a psychiatrist finally rescued him from his "cardiac neurosis."

Sir James Mackenzie closed his medical office on Harley Street in London one day and returned to the small country town in Scotland where he was born. His interests had turned, increasingly, to the study of the "normal" in human beings and how to maintain it—the practice of true preventive medicine. In London he had found that patients who consulted him were too often beyond repair. Now he hoped to answer the compelling question: What were the bad habits that led to disease?

After a rich life of practice and intelligent observation, he arrived at three conclusions:

(1) Diseases are the result of long-developing processes which begin early in life and finally lead to saturation of the body with toxins.

(2) Improper eating, living and thinking habits are the prime cause of this degeneration.

(3) The same type of toxin when localized in a joint causes arthritis; when localized in the liver, hepatitis; in the kidneys, nephritis; in the skin, dermatitis; in the pancreas, diabetes; in the brain, insanity.

But the bulk of Dr. Mackenzie's illuminating published observations dealt with heart damage, which be believed resulted from the same toxin. His conclusion was that the heart is troubled all too often by a chemical disturbance of the body, and my own observations with heart patients confirm this theory. Where the heart is not too badly damaged, recovery always follows after the chemical disturbance is removed.

11

Defects in Kidneys and
Blood Pressure

When Shakespeare wrote, "A man of my kidney," he used it as a term of admiration, for he considered the kidneys as organs of courage and high quality. But in the prim days of Queen Victoria the kidneys, as part of the excretory function, were never mentioned in polite society.

Today we are less squeamish; yet our kidneys, like our livers, are greatly insulted internal organs. Man, ignorant of the chemistry and functions of the kidneys and the liver, constantly mistreats both by undue strain as a consequence of dietetic errors. He refers to his kidneys as being "sluggish" and resorts to advertised kidney or liver pills as a palliative. Or he attempts to whip them with drugs and other stimulants, or he tries to remedy the situation by flooding them with copious draughts of water.

The much abused kidneys are among the most complex organs in the body; I am continually amazed when I observe how patiently they bear up under duress; how tirelessly and valiantly they strive to do their work, never letting up for one minute; never behaving in a slothful manner. Even when literally burned up with poisons, they labor heroically, until finally overwhelmed by toxemia. Uremic poisoning and congestive heart failure, due to terminal-stage kidney disease, is the nation's fourth-ranking cause of death—over a hundred thousand people a year.

Like physicians, engineers and mechanics are best able to appreciate the kidneys as marvelous filtering devices. Although small enough to fit into the palm of your hand, each kidney is equipped with a million individual filter units. Each kidney, too, can filter seventeen hundred quarts of viscous fluid in twenty-four hours. There are some fifty different chemicals dissolved in this liquid. The kidneys, after determining which ones are needed in the body, reabsorbs them and filters out the unneeded ones.

The structure of the kidney is not only beautifully designed for its work but exceedingly fascinating to study. Yet it is simple to understand. There are two of these remarkable little organs, shaped like the bean named after them, which lie in the back, just under the diaphragm, their upper poles covered by the last two or three ribs. About four or five inches long, two and a half inches wide and one and a half inches thick, the kidney feels solid, weighs as much as an orange and is exquisitely designed to perform its work as the "great purifier" of the body. The kidney's chief blood supply is from arteries that branch from the large main artery which descends from the heart. The adrenal glands lie against the upper poles of the kidneys, perched on them like caps.

Three divisions are seen in the cross section of a kidney. An outer zone is a dark red color and is about half to three quarters of an inch wide. This division contains the tiny globes, each at the end of a small artery (arteriole). These globes filter water from the blood. The middle division is lightest in color and consists of a meshwork of fine tubules, surrounded by minute veins (venules). These tubes carry the water, which has been filtered, to a central drainage area. The third or inner division, which is called the pelvis of the kidney, is a reservoir which drains through a long tube (ureter) into the bladder. The first two divisions contain no sensory nerves and thus cannot register pain when disordered; the kidney pelvis is lined with cells richly supplied with sensory nerves that register pain from kidney stones or excessive acidity or alkalinity of the urine. Also similarly equipped and also sensitive are the ureter and bladder.

The kidney's main blood supply is arterial—the cleanest, reddest blood in the body. It will be remembered that the blood supply of the liver is almost entirely venous—the most impure, bluish blood of the body. Snugly encased in a strong, inelastic capsule of fibrous tissue, the kidney is embedded in a cushion of fat, thus protected from physical harm.

Many people think of the kidney as merely part of the body's garbage-disposal unit. But because of the kidney, man was able, in the words of Dr. Homer W. Smith, to transform himself "from fish to philosopher."

The kidney originated when water-breathing creatures like the fishes became air-breathers and moved from water to dry land. Fishes, surrounded by water in the salty warm sea, maintained a certain concentration of water in their tissues, absorbed and excreted by their gills much the same as the concentration of air in our bodies is regulated by the lungs. When certain ancient fish finally developed lungs and became air-breathers, a new blood-water balance had to be maintained. For this purpose the kidney evolved.

It is, therefore, an automatic regulator which keeps the water in the blood and body tissues at about the same mildly salty concentration as that found in fish. The blood serum contains salts identical to those found in sea water, and so body cells are still literally bathed in the sea. Thus, in our process of evolution, we have never wandered far away from the protection of a sea mother. So, too, each new life spends its first nine months within the womb's mothering sea.

Water is introduced into the body by drinking or by eating foods with a high water content (vegetables, fruits, meats, milk) or originates from the metabolism of sugars, starches and fats. As sugars and starches or fats are metabolized, they are gradually oxidized to their end products, which consist of carbon dioxide and water (CO_2 and H_2O). This water is called *metabolic water* and is often reabsorbed and used in the body while the carbon dioxide is eliminated through lung exhalation. Thus is the body's water balance maintained.

The function of metabolic water is well illustrated in the life habits of the bull seal. In the spring, an enormously obese creature, he swims to the spawning grounds on the rocky coasts of the northern seas. There he stakes off ground for his expected harem and guards this enclosure from other bulls with his best fighting strength. About a month later the females arrive. He gathers his "wives," attacks other bulls who encroach upon his domain and fertilizes his females. Then, three to four months later, he swims south, thin, weak, bruised, battered and anemic from bleeding wounds. During his stay at the spawning grounds he neither eats nor drinks, though he regularly passes urine. His water supply comes from metabolic water, one of the end products of fat oxidation.

Another example is the antelope of the Mexican desert who drinks no water for a very good reason—there is none in his domain. This hearty creature obtains his water from cacti and other plants and from his own metabolic water. During the hottest part of the year, a period of from nine to ten months, he passes no urine at all, for his urine is absorbed to maintain his water balance. The same happens to his neighbor the kangaroo rat. Thus, no matter how hot or dry the climate, some creatures can live without drinking water.

The food in man's natural diet contains enough water for his needs; thus, it should be generally unnecessary for him to drink water. What, then, makes us thirsty? The desire comes after the ingestion of salt, condiments, sweets and concentrated starches, which are usually eaten in a dry state. Fruits and vegetables, especially when eaten raw, contain from 70 to 90 percent water; milk as high as 85 percent; meat 50 to 60 percent. The quality of water found in melons, papayas, raw carrots, cucumbers and celery is distinctly more beneficial to the body than the chlorinated, chemically processed and irritating fluid that too often comes from the faucet.

One of the chief functions of the kidney is to rid the blood of excessive water. Metabolic water is one of the two end products of carbohydrate metabolism; the other is carbon dioxide gas, which is eliminated through the lungs.

The filtration of water through the tiny globes of the kidney is dependent upon blood with a high oxygen content, so arterial blood —richest in oxygen—is used. But when the arterial blood contains abnormal impurities, due to improper diet, the kidneys need *extra* oxygen to force elimination; this extra oxygen is supplied by the adrenal glands. Nature wisely placed these glands near the kidneys, so that their internal secretion (adrenoxidase) can supply oxygen faster, in order to overcome any strain on the process taking place in the globule of the kidney. As I have noted earlier, the abnormal diet of civilized man throws extra work upon his adrenals. Thus, the hard-working adrenals help to facilitate elimination of waste products through the kidneys, but this additional task tends to deplete the adrenal glands and perhaps shorten the individual's life.

There are many drugs and food toxicants which, by stimulating the adrenals, force impurities from the blood via the kidneys. This temporary blood cleansing often produces remarkable results. Naturally the patient as well as the doctor is pleased with miracles.

For instance, not so long ago, newspapers were full of exciting pictures showing an arthritic cripple throwing away his crutches. Toxic products, which had been irritating the joints (rheumatism), were more rapidly eliminated by the kidneys after dosing the patient with the wonder drug cortisone. But the last act of this vaudeville show was not pictured in the papers. The same patient, his adrenals exhausted from the overstimulation, lay victimized by advanced arthritis as well as drug poisoning.

Another rather absurd idea about the kidneys is based upon the observation that the more water taken, the more urine there is passed. The bottled-water companies exhort the public to drink eight glasses a day. Then there are the elaborate and expensive spas, here and abroad, where poisons can be temporarily flooded out of the body. People believe they can eat, drink and be merry for eleven and a half months a year, and then spend two weeks renewing themselves before starting the cycle afresh.

There is a catch in it, though. Neither the sweat glands nor the kidneys can eliminate a great quantity of toxins from the blood over a short period of time without great strain or damage to the heart. Thus the concentration of these poisons is always maintained in the blood at a low level. After five minutes of intense sweating, or thirty minutes after excessive water drinking, *no toxic compounds* can be found either in the sweat or urine. There is only a clear and colorless secretion which is nothing but water. It takes about twenty-four hours before the toxin content of the blood rises enough to make another such elimination possible. Therefore, a short sweat, or a small increase of drinking water daily, will do the patient more good, with less strain on the body's temperature mechanism and less load on the heart, than a continual dousing, which makes it necessary to push all these excess fluids around the body. It is known that sudden deaths after the administration of intravenous fluids and blood transfusions result from inability of the heart to pump the overload of fluids.

About 90 percent of the benefit to the patient taking spa treatment comes from mental relaxation, vacation change and rest, even though the diet is often atrocious at these places. Too, many are very expensive. A week's rest at home, fasting on fruit and vegetable juices and bathing frequently in a tub of warm water to which Epsom salts and Glauber's salts have been added, will accomplish more good with much less drain on the purse and less strain on the kidneys. This same treatment will also lower an elevated blood pressure.

A medical term which has gained great popularity and is frequently used by the healing profession is the word "dehydration." Next to the dread "cancer," it evokes a powerful sense of fear in the mind of the patient. When thoroughly frightened, a sick man will submit to an unlimited quantity of fluid injected into his veins. As with the water cure, this extra fluid is supposed to dilute and wash away toxic material. The most popular mixture contains glucose (sugar), which is supposed to feed the starving cells of the body, and normal salt solution. Laboratory tests on animals show, however, that intravenous glucose is stored in the liver, spleen, and other internal organs and is never oxidized as food. The salt solution is often retained in the tissues and appears to lessen the state of dehydration, but actually it fails to accomplish much permanent good. The patient's appearance is improved much the same as the looks of a corpse are improved when the sunken tissues are filled with embalming fluid.

When a body is too weak to absorb fluids naturally, it is too weak to live. If the fluids cannot be retained by mouth, due to nausea and vomiting, they can be given by rectum. The large bowel's ability to absorb water into the system is even greater than that of the stomach. Water given in this manner will be accepted or rejected by the body as it desires, and it is never "forced" to take it. Fluids are absorbed slowly by rectum. Of course, this method takes time and patience on the part of the nurse or attendant; it is so much quicker and easier to give it intravenously, but with the IV method there is always an element of risk to the patient, due to excessive strain on the heart or kidneys. Instead of suffering from dehydration, the patient may be in a state of inanition and should be treated in a different manner. But at present, "IVs" are in fashion, for, like Paris gowns, medical fashions come and go.

We may well question what *really* beneficial effect intravenous solutions have on moderately advanced cases of kidney trouble and high blood pressure. Occasionally, perhaps, there is temporary help, as long as the adrenal glands are strong enough to respond. Working as one of the most powerful defense mechanisms of the body, these glands react against sudden changes in blood volume. The additional adrenal secretion stimulates the kidneys to increased function, facilitating toxic elimination. But the tired horse can never be whipped too long before finally lying down for good. If any benefit follows such treatment, it is of short duration and may do more harm than good.

Much has been written in popular publications concerning blood pressure and, indeed, it is also a very lively topic in medical circles. Great effort has been directed toward lowering the pressure, and practically every new wonder drug has been tried. The popular belief is that all abnormal states, such as fever, pain, nervousness, etc., should be done away with, the quicker the better. But to understand blood pressure, one must look carefully into the heart and kidney function.

The globule of the filtration apparatus of the kidney has already been described. A normal, healthy person has about a million globules in each kidney. Experiments on animals have shown that complete health can be maintained on one fourth of the total kidney substance, and that under such circumstances the animal's blood pressure remains normal. Roughly, in this case, the filtration is then being done by 250,000 globules. When there is a steady chemical destruction of globules, elevation of blood pressure begins. To simplify and illustrate the problem, smaller digits can be used: suppose twenty globules can filter one unit of blood in two minutes, with the body remaining in a healthy state; if ten globules are destroyed, one unit of blood cannot circulate for filtration in two minutes unless twice the volume of blood is driven through the ten globules; to drive twice the volume through, the pressure must be elevated, and the heart, if it is a good strong organ, elevates the pressure by beating harder; the adrenal glands supply the tone and energy the heart needs to accomplish this feat, and this extra adrenal secretion in the blood simultaneously enhances the globule function of the kidney.

From this illustration it can be understood that elevation of blood pressure is an emergency measure to help the patient and that the *cause* of this high blood pressure is the *result* of kidney impairment. But with weak or exhausted adrenals no elevation of pressure is possible.

The questions now arise: What poison destroys the globules; where does it come from? We must remember that the kidney is an organ whose function is to maintain the water balance in the blood, water consumed by mouth and metabolic water. In every oxygen-breathing mammal, bird or reptile, such is the case. When the diet is proper, the *liver* eliminates the waste products of metabolism. It is only when the liver is unable to filter the blood properly that the kidneys are forced into a function they were never intended to perform. But in performing this function, the globules are gradually destroyed, so that presently both the liver and the kidneys degenerate.

Although it has long been known that high blood pressure was in some way related to impaired kidney function, it was not definitely and scientifically demonstrated until the remarkable experiments performed in the thirties by Dr. Harry Goldblatt of Cleveland. In his researches Dr. Goldblatt proved three things: (1) that the blood pressure became elevated when there was an interference with the rate of blood flow through the kidneys; (2) that this elevation of pressure was possible only when the adrenal glands were able to perform emergency duty; (3) that once the state of high blood pressure was produced, none of the commonly used remedies for lowering it were efficacious. In performing this most valuable, simple and irrefutable experimental work, Dr. Goldblatt merited high reward, yet his monumental work seems to have been overlooked; very few practicing doctors have even heard of it.

Dr. Goldblatt's experiments proved that elevated blood pressure results from the interference of blood circulation through the globules. The globules that have been destroyed by disease retard blood circulation. Nature elevates the pressure to insure sufficient blood supply through the remaining globules, and this restores the function of the kidneys. In his experiments, mostly on dogs, Dr. Goldblatt was able to cause the same amount of interference of blood flow simply by partially clamping the renal artery. When the caliber of the artery was thus reduced, blood pressure had to be increased in order for the kidney to have an adequate circulation. This was proved by the experiments, which also proved that the adrenal glands, controlling muscular tone (in the heart muscle as well as the contracting muscles of the artery walls), made this rise in blood pressure possible.

These remarkable experiments proved beyond a doubt that the rauwolfia group of drugs used, discarded and again accepted as specifics for high blood pressure, were completely ineffective. When there is an understanding of the relation of improper diet to the underlying toxemia which destroys the kidney globules, Dr. Goldblatt's experiments can be readily understood.

The most common irritants that cause a degeneration of the globules are salt, toxic protein acids (resulting from protein indigestion), metals (as mercury) and drugs. The resultant urine is composed mostly of pure water, since the weakened kidneys are unable to secrete the usual electrolytes (salts) and toxins.

It will be remembered that the globules normally secrete only water and the tubules conduct this water to the bladder for elimination. But just as the globules can become diseased by improper chemistry, so also can the tubules be destroyed. However, before tubular pathology can be understood, a word is necessary concerning tubular physiology. The function of the tubule is to conduct the water from the globule to the bladder. These tubules are able to reabsorb water if it is needed to maintain a normal balance in the body cells. The tubules are long, in order to give plenty of surface for reabsorption; they are also surrounded by a minute network of veins. When these veins contain diffusible acids resulting from improper digestion or oxidation of sugars and starches, the toxic elements can diffuse from the veins into the water of tubules and cause severe injury. Either acute or chronic tubular disease may result. In acute disease, we find blood and much albumen in the urine. If the tubules should be completely destroyed, anuria (stoppage of urine) results, followed rapidly by death.

In chronic disease varying amounts of albumen, red cells and casts are found. The casts are composed of the lining cells of the tubules. They can be clear or hyaline (gelatin-like), fine or coarsely granular, waxy or bloody. As the toxins trickle downward through the tubule (nephron), the concentration of toxic material increases. At the tubule's end, or what is called the lower nephron, the toxins can become so concentrated that they destroy the lower nephron and can, in fact, even terminate life. This condition is diagnosed as a lower nephron nephrosis, and is often seen in medical practice. When a patient becomes toxic, globules as well as tubules can be involved in a destructive process; therefore it is unusual to see either a purely globular or purely tubular nephrosis.

The tubule, although of great length (it is said that each kidney contains over a mile of tubules), is lined with a single layer of thin cells. The veins are also thin, the result being that diffusion easily takes place from one to the other. When the diffusible substance, always foreign, is toxic, great harm results. Not only does the diffusible toxin irritate and finally destroy the kidney tubule; it can also diffuse from the veins into the lymphatic vessels (there are many miles of these in the body) and be temporarily or permanently stored there as edema, commonly known as dropsy.

Sometimes the toxic material in the veins (due to imperfect filtration of the venous blood by the liver, itself damaged by toxins) reaches a high enough concentration to cause an inflammation of the vein itself. The blood in this part of the vein often clots; the resultant catastrophe is known as phlebitis. The clot may break loose and go floating around in the circulation to plug up the opening of a blood vessel, resulting in what is called an infarct. This plugging of the vessel causes an anemic area in the region supplied by the plugged vessel and often a necrosis, or death, of that area also. Through a careful study of the urine the character of the toxemia can be determined, often long before great destruction has been done. Then a curative diet can be prescribed which gradually relieves the kidney of the burden of forced vicarious elimination.

The earliest treatment for kidney disease was based on the premise that dilution was better than concentration. Intake of liquids, such as water, soups or juices, was pushed to the limit, thus coaxing the kidneys to eliminate toxins more rapidly in diluted form. Since many of the urinary poisons were acids the prescribing of alkalis as antidotes became popular. When the patient could not drink sufficient liquid to please his doctor, the fluid was given subcutaneously, intraperitoneally or intravenously. Forty-five years ago Dr. Martin H. Fischer, eminent physiologist and colloid chemist at the University of Cincinnati, was using a mixture of alkaline salts, mainly baking soda, to dehydrate edematous tissues and neutralize acids in cases then called nephritics.

With the exception of NaCl and certain poisonous drugs, the chief kidney irritants, according to my research, originate from improper digestion of proteins, carbohydrates or hydrocarbons. But to facilitate diagnosis, complicated kidney-function tests are not needed. They can do more harm than good because they contain aniline dyes and other irritants and foreign poisons that add to the impairment of the kidney function. The most practical kidney-function test is based on an assay of the urine after protein, sugar, starch or fat feeding. How do the kidneys behave after such test meals? What is the effect on blood pressure, on edema, on the heart?

Let me cite an example from my files of how I treated a case of hypertension, or high blood pressure. The patient was symptomless except for a slight shortness of breath after exertion; the blood pressure was 260/110. The urine was clear, light, with a fixed specific gravity of 1010. No edema was present. The history of the patient disclosed the fact that he had consumed far too much protein during most of his life. I prescribed bed rest and a diet consisting mainly of dietetic antidotes. The following alkaline elements in the form of vegetable broths were then prescribed: sodium chloride, sodium carbonate, sodium phosphate, sodium iodide, sodium fluoride, sodium bromide, sodium silicate and sodium borate (in vegetables, these minerals are all found in organic form). Potassium was given in similar combinations; calcium or calcium carbonate, chloride and phosphate; iron as chlorophyll compounds. Many trace elements and vitamins are always present in the above. Remember, this is not a "diet"; it is a *therapy*, consisting of useful, non-irritating and antidotal elements, all organic in nature.

In general such patients are kept at rest from five to seven days. If the blood pressure has dropped to 120/80, a common occurrence by then, we know that the hypertension was the result of an inflammatory state of the globules, which, not being irreparably damaged, quickly returned to normal function as a result of the antidote therapy. But suppose that after from five to seven days there was a drop to 210/110. We may then assume that there had been a great deal of globular damage which was irreversible. This is a practical, harmless kidney-function test.

A female patient presented herself complaining of edema (another case from my files). Examination showed dropsy of hands, legs and face. The circumference of her legs was three times what was normal for her. She felt waterlogged and her limbs were heavy. For years she had been a cream eater, using half-and-half in coffee, enjoying sour cream, ice cream and cream cheeses. The damage to the kidneys clearly was due to hydrocarbons (fats). Her urine was bile-colored, dark, thick; many casts were present. This was a case of "lower nephron nephrosis." In three weeks the urine was clear and all edema had disappeared. Fats, especially cream and butter, had been forbidden and the only carbohydrate allowed was raw cane sugar. The diet contained necessary amounts of protein (not over-cooked) and an excess of the required antidotes, in this case consisting mainly of raw and stewed fruits and vegetables. Later the patient determined by experiment just how much cream she was able to use without the return of the edema and dark urine. This was a practical, harmless kidney-function test.

Another example: a good adrenal type, a farmer of Swedish descent, was bedridden for six months because of massive edema of the legs (so great that he could not bend at the waist), free water (ascites) in the abdomen (at least one to two gallons), and water at the bases of both lungs (pleural effusion). He had been treated for two years, but no attention was paid to his diet. His face was so edematous it resembled a pumpkin and his eyes were lost in the bottom of deep cracks. Scarcely any urine was passed. When examined, his urine contained four-plus albumen and much pus and it was extremely amber-red in color. This man had been a heavy starch eater all of his life, enjoying three or four kinds at every meal. His blood pressure was 200/120 and the stethoscope revealed pronounced cardiac effort. But he was a tough Swede. He was placed on diluted grapefruit juice only, and his bowels were washed out twice a day with 20-percent-milk enemas. Soon his urine began to clear and in two weeks he had lost forty-five pounds of dropsy; his blood pressure had gone down to 120/90. Three weeks later he was doing his spring plowing. This patient remained in good health for the following twenty years by greatly restricting his starch intake. Again, an instance of a practical and harmless kidney-function test.

It is often impossible to determine the functional ability of the kidney until practical tests, synonymous with proper treatment, have been performed. The kidneys as well as the liver may show pathological injuries due to toxic protein or carbohydrate or hydro-carbon products. Amelioration of distressing symptoms always follows antidotal diet, providing the functional capacity has not been too greatly crippled by atrophy resulting from toxemia. Instead of compelling impaired kidneys to function by whipping the adrenal glands with drugs, a therapy based upon a natural treatment is suggested—one which removes the cause by prescribing an organic chemical therapy. As the late Dr. Alexis Carrel warned us, natural health is quite different from the state of unnatural stimulation, even though, to the unpracticed eye, it looks the same.

12

Your Weight: Too High or Too Low?

There are two classes of society that are extremely pitiable—fat people trying to get thin and thin people trying to get fat. Hundreds, perhaps thousands, of books have been written on cures for obesity, yet very few people successfully get rid of this disease. Any physician will tell you the melancholy fact that in the battle of the bulge, it is safe to say that old devil appetite is still far ahead of both the doctor's warnings and the drug laboratories' concoctions of painless reducing products.

All over the country "reducing diets" are a popular topic of conversation, yet few people lose weight permanently. The public has been warned over and over again that obesity is the nation's most serious health problem, yet physicians still find it one of the most difficult of all diseases to treat. Our fattened pocketbooks and our social mores contribute to the difficulty; calorie-rich peanuts and potato chips, cheese dips and alcoholic drinks at most social gatherings, doughnuts at "coffee breaks" and candy and sugar-rich soft drinks at hand throughout the day.

Patients frequently do lose weight for a while, but they tend to backslide and put it right on again. A cycle of overeating, gaining ten pounds, going on a crash diet and taking it off, then stepping right on the merry-go-round again is even more hazardous than remaining overweight. There is evidence now that this seesawing may be one of the causes of high blood pressure, doing damage to the blood vessels.

Dieting, when necessary, is a lifetime process. If you plan to lose weight, then you must be certain that you will keep it off.

Considering the enormous number of books, magazine and newspaper articles that have failed to make any appreciable dent in the thousands of obese persons, I approach the subject with a good deal of hesitation. But my findings on obesity go beyond the commonly accepted, easy-on-the-doctor method of handing out a printed low-calorie diet to the diet-conscious patient. Nor does my treatment for underweight consist of the nonsensical advice to feed the patient vast quantities of rich desserts and starchy foods.

There are two general types of obese persons. The Falstaffian, roly-poly, adrenal-type individual—happy, food-loving and hardly inconvenienced by his rotundity. The second type worries about his obesity as a threat to health and appearance and is desperately anxious to find an "easy" way to lighten his burden; he disdains the *hard* way, which is a drastic cutting of calories, and he is forever in search of some panacea—diet food, pill, oil, wafer, vinegar, etc.—to do the job for him.

There are, in my opinion, only two ways to reduce weight:

(1) *through total fasting, which is not eating at all, but drinking as much water as wanted;*
(2) *by special diets, based on the patient's needs.*

Recently newspaper and magazine articles have been stressing the value of fasting for weight reduction as though it were a newly discovered therapy. But there is nothing new about total fasting—the Old and New Testaments mentioned it seventy-four times; Hippocrates used the method. Through the years it has been widely used, then neglected. Mark Twain, in one of his articles, admitted he gained a reputation as a doctor by merely telling his sick friends to do what he did: "fast for forty-eight hours." At the present time certain members of the medical profession are again recommending controlled hospital fasting for those who fail to reduce by the usual methods. Results are dramatic, effective, as the pounds melt away. But total fasting can be, and often is, a dangerous method of weight reduction unless the cases are carefully selected, supervised in a hospital by a physician who thoroughly understands the fasting technique. An unsupervised do-it-yourself fast of more than two days should never be attempted.

Here is where the danger lies: *when an obese person begins the fast, it is tremendously important to know whether his overweight is normal fat or a state of toxic bloat.*

In the first case, the fast on distilled water is generally well tolerated, extremely beneficial, and results in much weight loss as the patient burns up his excess fat for nourishment. The pounds literally pour off at the rate of approximately two and a half a day; later there may be a loss of a pound a day. Generally there is some hunger for the first two days; then the craving disappears. I have known patients to lose twenty-five pounds in a ten-day total fast. These dramatic results, painlessly achieved, are of tremendous help to the chronically overweight (intractably obese) patient when other methods, such as limiting calories, do not work.

In the second case, where there is a state of toxic bloat, the fast may precipitate an acute toxic crisis, which may do the patient infinite harm or even lead to his destruction.

During the fast, the liver acts solely as an instrument of elimination. Quantities of waste products are discharged into the alimentary canal. It is this toxic bile, when reabsorbed, which causes havoc during the fast, especially when the patient's obesity is due to a toxic bloat. This "elimination crisis," with diarrhea, vomiting, weakness and serious dehydration, is often observed.

All this shows that fasting is not a medical toy to be played with, fascinating though it is. Great care must attend the fasting treatment. And though remarkably effective in treating obesity with disease complications, total fast is not to be used indiscriminately for self-indulgent patients who *do* respond to limiting calories. But for those with intractable obesity, it is worth considering that the patient did not get into his abnormal condition overnight; that it was months, possibly years, developing. The safest method to follow, therefore, is a gradual process of elimination and detoxication through short repeated fasts which do not place an undue strain upon delicate and damaged organs. Most fasters do suffer from weakness and should have bed rest or limited exercise. One over-weight doctor, among fifty-seven patients on a controlled total fast, had this to say: "This is a fine way to get the ball rolling, since no other program helped me. After the fast, it's easier to embark on a long-range plan I can live with, taking just enough food for my daily needs." (The second method of weight reduction, that of special diets, I'll discuss later in connection with cases from my files.)

There have been about as many changes in fashion in treating obesity as in ladies' hats. In 1888 *The Relation of Alimentation and Disease*, by Dr. James H. Salisbury, attracted much attention. Dr. Salisbury was one of the first observers to connect obesity with sugar and starch eating; he cured his patients by corrective diet, consisting of meat, vegetables and fruits—a very up-to-date reducing diet. With it he not only successfully cured obesity but also a long list of other diseases including arthritis and tuberculosis. It was his opinion that the fermentation of starches gave rise to the formation of vinegar (acetic acid); he was able to repeat the disagreeable symptoms following heavy starch intake by simply giving vinegar to his patients.

One of the harmful effects of vinegar in the human body is that it tends to leach out the body's phosphorus and also stimulate the thyroid gland. As the phosphorus becomes depleted, the adrenal function diminishes, since phosphorus is one of the active components of the adrenal secretion. Salisbury observed so many disagreeable and dangerous symptoms by the ninth day in his experimental subjects on the vinegar diet that he was forced to terminate the experiment. These symptoms included headache, throat congestion, mucus expectoration, pains in the heart, sour perspiration, alternate fever and chills and rapid pulse. The patients did lose weight because of the induced hyperthyroidism and the hypo-adrenalism. Even as far back as forty years ago vinegar was recommended to keep the body slim and was popularly used by young women. There are cases on record which show that this treatment undoubtedly caused tuberculosis by this chain of events. Acetic acid (vinegar), neutralized by the phospholecithins of the blood serum, resulted in a toxic ester forming tubercles in the lungs. Germs fed on and broke down the tubercles. The germs did not cause tuberculosis—they acted as scavengers. Vinegar is a waste product of the body and may be found at times in the urine. In small doses it is stimulating and in cases of toxemia from heavy starch intake it may have somewhat the same neutralizing effect as citrus juices. But for reducing it should be avoided.

Dr. Salisbury was followed by Horace Fletcher, who believed that if you chewed each mouthful of food until it "slipped unconsciously down the throat," you would not only benefit but would lose weight because you ate less. Most dieters do eat too fast; if they ate more slowly, they would feel more satisfied.

Later, a number of doctors, notably Dr. Blake F. Donaldson, advocated a total meat diet for obesity as well as for many other diseases. But what Dr. Donaldson fails to do with his high-protein diet (according to my investigations) is to realize that people suffering from certain protein injuries of the liver may be poisoned by excess protein. He fails also, I think, to realize that fat injuries can lead to boils, carbuncles and other skin diseases resulting from toxic fatty acids. There is no doubt that the "high-protein or total-protein" diet does make for rapid weight loss, but it may leave other ills in its place. And so I do not recommend it.

When people who eat quantities of meat, in order to reduce or merely because they like meat, come to me for treatment, I cannot take them off their meat diet immediately, for they could not get along—they would just collapse. They have leaned on the high acidity of their meat diet so entirely that it is their main prop. When I have a case so far saturated, I must be most careful how I withdraw that item from their diet. With over-proteinized patients, I usually do not even touch the protein side of the diet for the first six months; I try to increase vegetables and vegetable soups to see what I can flush out before I start to take away meat. (A fuller discussion of this subject is found in the chapter "Proteins Can Be Body Killers.")

Although I cannot agree with Dr. Donaldson's total meat diet, I do heartily concur in his criticism of monosodium or mono-

potassium glutamate, a flavor enhancer for cooking, highly advertised under various trade names. In *Strong Medicine* Dr. Donaldson
says:

> The safest rule is not to buy anything that contains it. Whole
> cookbooks are written around the ability of monosodium
> glutamate to "flavor food." Instead of flavoring, what it does
> is to irritate the wall of the stomach to a stage of bright red
> acute congestion. The acute congestion causes a hunger sensa-
> tion, so you ask for a second helping. The Japs sent shiploads
> of it to us before the last war in exchange for our scrap steel,
> and now great factories in this country perpetrate it upon the
> public. Most of the canned soup that you buy contains the
> miserable stuff. Manufacturers aren't particularly bright when
> they listen to their chemists. When the public realizes that
> acute congestion of the stomach is an almost ideal way to in-
> duce cancer in that organ in a susceptible individual, canned
> soups will change their ways.

I, too, have observed that monosodium glutamate, besides irritating the taste buds of the tongue and thereby enhancing food flavors,
also stimulates the thyroid gland and speeds up the heart. This, of
course, would have a tendency to make the patients lose weight and
is similar in its effect to thyroid extract.

Curtailing the diet has never been popular with the public as a
means of losing weight. Many people, through lifelong habit, are
addicted to certain amounts of food and they do not feel well and
contented unless their stomachs are full. So the possibility of allowing them to eat satisfying quantities and adding agents to the diet
which would interfere with the absorption of nourishment offered
itself as a means of circumventing obesity.

About forty years ago Sir W. Arbuthnot Lane, noted consulting
surgeon to Guy's Hospital, London, became interested in chronic
intestinal intoxication and constipation. In his attempt to find mild,
non-irritating laxatives he experimented with various oils and finally
decided upon the use of liquid petrolatum (mineral oil). He noted
a tendency for patients to lose weight while taking the oil. Many

obesity cures since that time have been based on the use of various oils in the diet, but since many of them were chemically irritating to the intestinal mucous membranes, only neutral, non-irritating oils were found to be useful.

Today Lane's work has been forgotten, but a new oil therapy has been widely popularized for weight reduction. Any diet plan which says that calories don't count is unscientific. For calories do count, emphatically. There are dangers involved in drinking large quantities of oils. There are dangers, too, in such fads as the Hollywood Eighteen Day Diet or the Rice Diet, in reducing wafers, pills or capsules, in appetite-appeasing pills and in the crash diet. The "combination" or "pairs" diet—lamb chop-and-pineapple, grapefruit-and-black coffee, bananas-and-skimmed milk—are not only poorly balanced but monotonous. A particularly harmful diet is the grapefruit-black coffee one. The high acidity of the grapefruit might leach the sodium out of the liver. I have seen grapefruit diets destroy all the teeth; continued long enough by foolish females, it can thoroughly leach all the calcium out of the body.

Books could be written on the many easy and popular "cures" for obesity throughout history. Each has contributed its part to the formation of a more rational approach to the solution of this problem. It is a *real* problem: today one in every five Americans is overweight and is getting fatter. Carrying pounds of useless flesh is definitely a hazard to survival and not merely a matter of appearance. As someone said, "The more bodily weight you carry around, the shorter time you'll likely have to carry it."

In my opinion, before a case of obesity can be treated, the patient must be classified. There are three general headings: (1) overindulgence of food; (2) endocrine origins; (3) toxic overweight.

The patients suffering simply from overindulgence of food are perhaps the most numerous of all. Here the logical program to follow is simply to curtail the amount of food eaten. But these patients are so used to getting up from the table with a comfortably full feeling that it is very difficult for them to curtail their overeating, and if they do, they find themselves eating between meals or raiding the refrigerator at midnight—all of which simply adds to their obesity. It is, therefore, essential *literally* to stuff them with food containing the *least* number of calories.

I recommend beginning the meal with a homemade (never canned) vegetable soup, followed by a large salad, so huge that they are practically filled up before the richer foods are served. The bountiful salad also has a tendency to relieve the constipation which causes these patients to absorb their foods over longer intervals of time. The coffee break, now written into many union contracts, is bad for weight watchers because of the doughnuts consumed. The modern cocktail party also offers too many caloric temptations. One needs will power, a quality in short supply in the obese.

If they *must* snack between meals or while watching TV, I suggest limited amounts of fresh or cooked fruits, never dried, which are too high in sugar. On this regime the weight loss will be gradual instead of spectacular. And it is this gradual weight loss which is so disheartening to scale-watchers. No healthful reducing diet can be magically quick in results. Nor can it be a punishing diet, because the obese person will soon tire of that and the pounds will pile up again. I have found that the best way to win the war of the expanding waistline is a slow and steady retreat. That is what an elderly patient of mine did.

When I first saw her in March, 1961, she was 75, weighed 138 pounds and complained of much fatigue. Her blood pressure was 210/100. She had been taking blood pressure pills which afforded little relief. She was taken off the pills and given food as follows. Early A.M.: hot water; breakfast: red clover tea, stewed fruit and a small dish of cooked cereal; lunch: rare beef or lamb, cooked non-starchy vegetables and a tablespoonful of mashed potato or hard squash with a half pat of butter; midafternoon: one variety of fruit, fresh or cooked; dinner: a large serving of zucchini or string beans, rare beef and a boiled potato the size of a golf ball; at bedtime: fruit or vegetable soup. This was an ample supply of food and she never complained of hunger. It was easy for her to remain on the diet, and when I last saw her, in June, 1964, her blood pressure was 130/70, her weight remained at 113 and she was symptom-free.

The second type, that of endocrine origin, presents a different problem. The most common kind of endocrine obesity is seen in the adrenal type of individual or among patients suffering from adrenal tumors, or simple enlargement of the adrenal glands. These patients seem to absorb nourishment more quickly than average persons and increase their weight on really very small amounts of food. Being adrenal types, they are naturally of the draft-horse build, square and muscular to begin with, and they are especially prone to gain fat from the ingestion of sugar, starches and fats—to which they usually are addicted. A diet consisting of lean meats, unsweetened drinks, fresh and cooked fruit, fresh and cooked non-starchy vegetables will be most beneficial—if they will stay on it. Cream, butter, eggs, meat fats and gravies must be avoided.

Exercise is extremely valuable in these cases—to preserve muscle tone and aid in oxidizing carbon compounds. But it must be started slowly and in an amount that is easy to perform, then advanced gradually, if they have previously spent "more time on the seat than on the feet."

One of my patients was a man with this adrenal type of obesity. He weighed 203 pounds and his blood pressure was 110/80. He had no complaints, merely wished to reduce to 165 pounds if possible. First seen in May, 1963, he was placed on a diet low in sugars and starches. By October, he weighed 180 after carefully following the diet. But after Thanksgiving and Christmas he was up to 197 and the following year in September he weighed 200 pounds. Although he eats very sparingly of sugars and starches, he is the typical adrenal type and it is probably impossible to reduce his weight permanently.

Another endocrine obesity type is seen in cases of thyroid-gland depletion, commonly known as myxedema, which is rather rare in this country. The average busy medical practitioner seldom sees more than half a dozen a year. When they can be cured, the cure depends upon the ingestion of thyroid extract or foods especially rich in iodine. Since those suffering from myxedema do not handle their starches well, it is best for them to omit all starchy foods from their diet. When their thyroid glands are not too deteriorated, miraculous transformations follow the taking of thyroid. Probably the indiscriminate use of thyroid extract for practically any kind of obesity, as well as for stimulative purposes, has arisen from its use in myxedematous cases. Much of this erroneous therapy is based upon misinterpreted basal metabolic rates or estimation of iodine in the blood. It must be remembered that minus basal rates depend not only on thyroid underactivity but also adrenal and liver impairment.

Many patients with liver impairment and weak adrenals have low basal rates, although their thyroids are hyperactive. These patients react very poorly to thyroid therapy, and they may be driven into nervous breakdowns or states of heart trouble from such treatment. When estimation of iodine in the blood (the protein-bound iodine, or PBI, test popular at the present time) is used to evaluate thyroid activity, it must be remembered that in the very process of neutralization of toxins, the iodine can become so tightly bound up with the toxic protein molecule that the test fails to reveal it. This would give the impression that the patient's thyroid was subnormal when, in reality, it was overactive, and again, great harm could be done by administering thyroid extract.

The treatment of the third form, toxic obesity, is one of the most difficult of all for the physician. Here the overweight is due to water and mucus retention in the lymphatic channels of the body, and really represents a sidetracking of poisons into these tissues. With their impaired liver and kidney functions, they cannot eliminate toxic material rapidly enough, so it is conveniently packed into the tissues and bloats them into a state of overweight. When these patients undergo fasts or remedial diets, the strain of digestion is taken off the liver and the kidneys and the patient suffers what is called an "elimination crisis." This often not only greatly frightens him but also discourages him from following the treatment. There is usually one type of food whose digestion is seriously impaired, thus resulting in this bloated condition. His liver may be sensitive to sugars, starches, fats, proteins, coffee, tea, chocolate, vinegar, salt or other condiments. The careful physician can often determine which food is incompatible and the cure depends upon restricting this food in the diet or eliminating it. Usually, too, these patients are likely to overindulge in the foods that are the most toxic to them, because of their stimulation value: what they crave the most, although it peps them up and makes them feel better, is gradually causing a fatal cirrhosis of the liver. When these patients are put on a forty-eight-hour fast, great quantities of the most offending toxin may be found in their urine. This gives the physician a lead to the formation of a diet for them. Such a diet seems almost magical in its early results. On a careful diet, these are the people who can lose ten pounds a week. What is lost is toxic bloat, mostly water collected around excess salt, toxins, etc.

When placed on a more normal food intake, these patients suffer terribly from lack of stimulation, become weak and exhausted, and often require bed rest. All of the distressing symptoms following the beginning therapy must be carefully explained to them before treatment is started. There is often much loss of bloat in their faces, and their kind friends, especially the fat ones, will tell them how dreadful they are looking. After this initial stage of weakness, though, as their liver function gradually repairs, normal energy will return, which is a far different condition from what they previously thought was health but was only a state of toxic stimulation.

This symptom complex (syndrome) was thoroughly understood and carefully described by Dr. Alexis Carrel in *Man, the Unknown*. Not only are people deceived by the false sense of well-being of a toxic-stimulating diet, but physicians, in general, have learned very little from the brilliant observations of the late Dr. Carrel.

When the patient with this type of toxic obesity becomes well on a remedial diet, it is absolutely necessary that the foods which are often called allergenic be restricted from his diet for the rest of his life. This is not hard for him to do because he feels so much better when eating the foods that completely agree with him.

A case from my files well describes this allergy to a particular food. A woman of sixty-four, a socialite, clubwoman and busy housewife, came to see me for weight reduction and chronic fatigue. At the age of nineteen, when she weighed ninety-nine pounds, she was given a drug by her doctor that was supposed to reduce what he thought was an overactive thyroid gland. Soon she weighed 122, probably correct for her at that age. She then married, became pregnant and in 1926, after the birth of her first child, weighed 180 pounds. She did not lose weight after her second child was born. During the subsequent years, she fluctuated between 165 and 180. She became my patient in 1957 when she weighed 165. There was definite evidence of starch indigestion with resulting bloat. On a starch-free diet her bloat disappeared and her weight dropped to 145 (ideal for her). Although warned not to, she ate sweetened starches in 1961 and twice in 1964. Each time she suffered heart attacks, the last one quite serious. She now lives on cooked and raw vegetables, mostly non-starchy, and rare beef and lamb with a little fruit. Her life continues to be busy and energetic. There is no evidence of toxic bloat at her present healthy weight of 145 and there are no heart symptoms.

Gaining weight is often as much of a problem as trying to fight the battle of the bulge. The thin race-horse type of person, who usually has an overactive thyroid gland and weak or underactive adrenals, often remains thin for years. No matter how he tries to gain weight, his thyroid literally burns up his food before he has an opportunity to deposit it as fat. Many times these people, hoping to fill out their bony contours, will stuff themselves with sugars and starches, which in themselves stimulate the thyroid, and after a heavy dinner and a night of much perceptible heartbeating, they awaken only to find that they have lost one or two pounds. Too, the overindulgence in fattening foods often results in an indigestion which prevents them from eating a normal amount of food of any kind. Many of them are often forced to gain weight by drinking large quantities of milk, but when the milk is reduced the weight gain vanishes too.

In the underweight, I have observed that the greatest dietary mistakes are made because people believe that stuffing always results in obesity. This may very well be the case on the farm where geese are held with their bills open and food poured down their throats. But this system does not work with humans, especially with those of the thyroid type, who are often deluged with cream and butter until they either become jaundiced or break out with boils and carbuncles. It is far better to let them go their own way, dietetically, eating what agrees with them. During middle age, the activity of their thyroids often subsides, and they gain weight and even become obese on their previous diets.

One of the characteristics of the thyroid type of individual, be he thin or fat, is the absence of hunger for breakfast. This is usually due to the ingestion of a heavy evening meal, which not only taxes the digestion, but also causes a bilious state with loss of appetite. This person awakens with a toxic-bile hangover and regains his chemical equilibrium if he skips breakfast. Should he skip his evening meal, plus his usual bedtime snack, the appetite for breakfast would return and he would be able to digest it. This fact was observed many years ago when, in 1900, Dr. James Hooker Dewey published a book on the "no breakfast plan," which was very popular in its day and helped a great many thyroid-type patients recover from dyspepsia and a state of underweight.

Other dieticians have recommended a "no dinner" plan, or at least a very light one. Nutritionist Adele Davis believes we should "Eat breakfast like a king, eat lunch like a prince, but eat dinner like a pauper." I have found that it is highly beneficial for the dyspeptic person to eat less and thereby gain back his health and weight. Occasionally patients are seen who were born with a liver impairment and whose thyroid glands, by oversecreting, relieve the liver condition through helping the process of detoxication, since the iodine fraction of the internal secretion of the thyroid gland is a powerful detoxicant. These people eat lightly, stay well, strong and healthy a long time but remain persistently thin.

But it is the overweight patients who fill the doctors' offices across the land. Too many of them are searching for a delicious way to lose weight—"a pill that makes pounds melt away magically while you enjoy all the food you want"—as the advertisements put it. Unfortunately for them, science has not discovered such a pill. The hard fact still remains, as poet Walter De La Mare wrote:

It's a very odd thing—
As odd as can be—
That whatever Miss T. eats
Turns into Miss T.

13

From Appendicitis to
Women's Ailments

In the final analysis, health depends upon the circulation of pure blood. The composition of the blood depends upon the food we eat—nothing else. If proper food is eaten, normal blood is generated. If the blood is normal, the liver, kidneys, heart and all other organs function as they should. Under these ideal conditions disease is practically impossible.

In this chapter I will mention, briefly, a number of diseases not discussed in other chapters and their treatment by proper diet.

APPENDICITIS

In appendicitis there are two types of inflammation: chronic or acute. In a chronic type of long duration, there may be slowly progressing symptoms. The onset of acute appendicitis is sudden and accompanied by nausea and vomiting, fever and severe abdominal pain. The victim is rushed to the hospital for a "life-saving" appendectomy.

But is it *always* a life-saving procedure?

Although immediate surgery is usually indicated, there are valid reasons why it is not always the best procedure following an acute attack. For example, it is difficult to drain an abscess surgically, especially if the patient is forced to lie on his back. Drainage tubes cause foreign-body irritation and may result in adhesions and an ugly scar. There is also the possibility, however small, that the patient may die of peritonitis after the operation. But because of the simplicity of the surgical procedure, the high percentage of recoveries and the common symptom of a simple "bellyache" in the region of the appendix, appendectomy has become, next to tonsillectomy, the most common of operative procedures. The surgeon who performs this simple cutting and stitching operation is looked upon as a savior because he is removing something harmful—routing out the offending organ to bring prompt and complete restoration of health.

But let us examine such surgery in detail. Today more than ever before, the pre-operative drugs, the complicated anesthetic, the heavy antibiotic dosage and other post-operative medication, together with the exorbitant cost of surgery and hospitalization all tend to make the skeptical patient wonder whether there could be a simpler, more efficient method. It is now well known that antibiotic drugs are not entirely harmless. Though they seem to perform miracles, in reality they often shorten the span of the patient's life. Unfortunately, too, the later aftereffects of modern drugs are seldom connected with their usage.

In what he calls "the unsalutary effects of the antibiotic age," Dr. Herbert Ratner, professor of preventive medicine and public health at Loyola University Medical School, tells of his admiration "for the tremendous advances in medicine, whether in heart surgery or brain surgery, in antibiotics and immunizing agents. . . . These advances are translatable in terms of large numbers of people who in many instances would otherwise be dead. My point is that we are accomplishing this but in such a way that we are also increasing morbidities and anxieties. We do much for the dying but less for the living, and in some instances we directly convert the living to the dead by therapeutic misadventure. Unfortunately, illnesses and deaths caused by drugs are not among the reportable diseases. We must be ready and willing to move in with the art of medicine when nature needs help and can be helped with the forceful and decisive use of drugs and other procedures, especially in life-threatening situations. But we also have to learn to keep our hands off in conditions that do not warrant the application of powerful and dangerous drugs, or the use of radical and risky surgery."

Every thoughtful physician is concerned with the risks in using the powerful and dangerous antibiotics. Dr. Franklin Bicknell, in *Chemicals in Food*, says: "Antibiotics such as penicillin, aureomycin, terramycin, etc., are being universally and indiscriminately used in medicine to control any and every kind of infection, however trivial. . . . This wholesale use of the antibiotics has had two serious drawbacks: bacteria are developing resistance to the antibiotics, and the patients are becoming sensitized or allergic to them." Particularly shocking is the amount of penicillin used to treat infections in cows. This enters the milk supply and causes severe reactions to milk consumers.

But let us return to surgery. There is no doubt that in *certain* cases surgery is necessary. And many a patient is frightened by thoughts of the consequences if surgery is not performed immediately. So the nonconformist doctor, reluctant to resort to surgery in every case of acute appendicitis, finds it difficult to convince a patient to try another form of treatment. Occasionally, the patient has been trying home remedies and has refused to call a doctor until general peritonitis has set in. Even then, if the pus is promptly drained surgically, his life may be saved.

I have always believed that with special care a case of ruptured appendix could be cured without surgery. Here is an example: The patient was a forty-six-year-old man, interested for years in a careful choice of natural food. Small in stature, he was well developed, not obese, and weighed 135 pounds. His wife and their two children, whose births I attended, were also my patients. All were on well-chosen diets and all were healthy. Both patients were teachers who often attended social dinners; it was at one of these that the husband made an unwise choice of food. On July 19, at a Mexican dinner, he ate a large portion of tamale pie and green salad heavy with mayonnaise, and topped this off liberally with ice cream.

About two A.M. he was awakened by a severe pain in his abdomen. His wife gave him enemas with good results, but the intensity of the pain increased. They both concluded that it was due to an acute indigestion. He remained in bed all day, and since he had no appetite, he merely sipped water. Enemas were repeated at four-hour intervals. He was very uncomfortable and had a temperature of 100, accompanied by much nausea and vomiting. This brought up not only the previous night's dinner but the contents of his small intestine as well. About forty-eight hours later the pain suddenly ceased and he felt much more comfortable, but his fever rose to 101 and his pulse was rapid and thready. It was then that I was called.

Strangely enough, the patient did not appear to be ill. In fact, he said he felt like getting up and going to work the next morning. His pulse of 120 to the minute, his temperature of 101 and his previous symptoms all pointed to an acute appendicitis. I concluded that the appendix had ruptured, after which the pain had ceased. Since he had had no medication, his symptoms were not masked by analgesic drugs. The last few enemas returned uncolored and all movement of gas in his intestines had stopped. "I don't want surgery," he said, "if it can be avoided." "Fine," I told him, "but you must consent to hospitalization and surgical consultation while I treat you without the use of drugs or the knife." He agreed.

The surgical consultant, a staff member of Bellevue Hospital and a graduate of Columbia University Medical School, a competent man of great experience and a good friend, was willing to stand by and make daily examinations with me while watching the progress of the patient. The first examination in the hospital, on July 23, showed a tender mass in the region of the appendix—a mass about the size of an orange, which could also be palpated by rectum. There was no indication of peristaltic activity (alternate waves of constriction and dilation in the alimentary canal). Enemas were useless and cathartics strongly contraindicated. The most careful auscultation of the abdomen disclosed no evidence of the slightest movement of intestinal gas. It appeared that nature, in her wisdom, had ordered a state of complete quiet and rest.

The patient had slight nausea only when he changed his position in bed; vomiting had ceased. He was satisfied with small pieces of ice by mouth; there was no desire for food. The white blood count was 20,000 with 96 percent polymorph cells, which indicated an abscess with localized pus. His blood pressure was 100/70 with no irregularity of heart action. There was no abdominal pain except on pressure. He slept well.

The following day, July 24, the nausea was negligible and pain on pressure was lessened. The patient was very comfortable in bed and enjoyed reading or listening to music. He also enjoyed small pieces of ice by mouth. I noted an abdominal mass the size of a grapefruit. The surgeon found the rectal mass larger and of more solid consistency.

On July 26, the white blood count had dropped to 12,000 with 85 percent polymorphonuclear leucocytes. (It is the white blood cells that act as policemen.) This was an indication that the abscess was well walled off and that there was less absorption of the toxins. The temperature had dropped to 99.6; the pulse to 90 and of fairly good strength. The blood pressure was 100/70. There was no nausea or vomiting. The consistency and size of the mass was the same.

Next day, the condition of the patient remained unchanged. There was not the slightest sign of peristalsis. A small, warm-water enema was given daily, and was returned uncolored and with no traces of feces.

When I visited him on July 27 he expressed a desire for grapefruit. The juice of a ripe grapefruit, diluted with two parts of water was given, along with small pieces of ice. The temperature remained at 99.6. There was no peristalsis and no pain, even on pressure. Yet the mass remained the same size. The patient was very comfortable, unfrightened and enjoyed his rest. My friend the surgeon was flabbergasted. I think he still entertained thoughts of draining the abscess. I believed that the abscess, although well walled off, would gradually "point" toward the adjacent wall of the large bowel, through which it would finally rupture and that there would be no peristalsis until the wall of the abscess broke and its contents were discharged into the large bowel. Then a putrid, blood-and-pus bowel movement would follow. This would occur from the twelfth to the fourteenth day after the onset of the attack.

There was no change the following day, July 28, except that the temperature had dropped to 99.

On July 29 there was still no evidence of peristalsis. The size of the mass remained the same. But the temperature dropped to 98.6; blood pressure to 90/60. The heart was regular with no cardiac exertion, the pulse 80. The patient remained satisfied on the diluted grapefruit juice and reported no craving for other foods. The white blood count was still 12,000 with 80 percent polys. The urine was negative, as it had been from the start. During the entire attack the only finding in the urine was an increase in the indican content (which meant that the putrefactive material was being absorbed into the blood from the bowel).

There was no change on July 30. The patient was not the least bit hungry. He was entirely satisfied with the grapefruit juice. The temperature was 98.5. The surgeon found conditions the same.

On July 31 the mass was smaller. The white blood count remained at 12,000, the polys had risen again to 85 percent. We were ready and impatient for the rupture of the abscess into the large bowel. The patient slept like a log at night and enjoyed several naps during the day. He looked thinner but healthier than ever. And he felt strong enough to do anything he cared to do. This included daily short strolls in the hospital corridor.

On August 1 the white blood count dropped to 11,000 with 83 percent polys; the blood pressure and pulse remained the same.

On August 2 the rupture finally occurred. The abscess mass was no longer palpable. The next morning there was a copious, spontaneous bowel movement which contained the contents of the abscess. The white count dropped to 8,000 with 80 percent polys. Now, for the first time, the patient developed an appetite. He weighed 110 pounds with blood pressure 100/60 and pulse normal at 70 beats to the minute. No mass was felt either by rectum or abdomen. At about six-hour intervals the patient continued to pass a small amount of fetid material from the bowel.

As his appetite increased the problem of desirable food presented itself. Other fruit juices were given, less diluted; also thin vegetable soups, carefully strained.

By August 5 he was drinking milk and eating egg yolks, cooked cereal, stewed ripe fruits and cooked non-starchy vegetables, such as string beans and soft squash. And he was discharged from the hospital. By September 12 he weighed 127 and was physically sound. Careful rectal examination showed no evidence of his former pathology.

One month later, he weighed 131, which I considered to be his normal weight. He was given a small dose of thyroid extract daily— one thirtieth of a grain—to help build up his thyroid gland, which had been depleted somewhat in its effort to detoxicate the body during the attack. This dosage was continued for about six months. Other than the thyroid the patient had no medication.

On July 21, when the appendix had ruptured and the acute pain disappeared, he was not exposed to heavy, deep palpation. Because of that, the pus from the broken appendix was not disseminated and no general peritonitis occurred. Once the appendix had ruptured, nature confidently built a wall around the fetid material and a localized peritonitis resulted, non-toxic to the patient because he was "properly treated." This proper treatment consisted of protecting the patient from well-meaning relatives who would have insisted on giving him "good nourishing food to keep up his strength." Had he been fed such food, even in small amounts, his fever would have mounted, his flatulence would have become unbearable, his pain would have increased, and his nausea and vomiting would have returned.

As treatment for this host of unfortunate conditions, large doses of sedative drugs might have been prescribed—drugs which could have paralyzed his sympathetic nervous system. This would have increased the abdominal gas to the point where "life-saving" surgery would have been necessary.

ASTHMA

Asthma is a catarrhal bronchitis involving the small bronchial tubes, including the smallest which are called bronchioles. This type of vicarious elimination is also under the control of the thyroid gland. The adrenal activity in asthma patients is much below normal, and because of this the chemistry of kidney function is impaired. Under duress, therefore, the lungs try to help the weak kidneys by secreting some of the toxins through their mucous membranes. But the lungs do not function well as accessory kidneys. Much inflammation results from the irritating toxins, with degeneration and atrophy of the bronchial tubes. Of all the organs in the body, the lungs are the most delicate; they can be severely damaged by any kind of irritant, be it tobacco smoke, smog or catarrhal inflammation. The chief toxins in asthma are sodium chloride and the toxic products of starch indigestion.

Many tests have shown that such treatment as ACTH, adrenalin and cortisone steroids have failed to cure asthma. But the elimination of all cereal grains, along with milk, egg, chocolate, fish and other less allergenic foods have brought relief to the asthma sufferer. I have found that definite poisonous substances can arise from starchy foods in the asthmatic's diet. Because fruit and other acid juices are irritating to the kidneys, it is dangerous to give them to the asthma patient during an attack, since in his case the fruit acids are incompletely oxidized in the liver.

The medical profession admits that there is no drug which will cure asthma. In fact, many doctors believe the disease to be incurable no matter what treatment is employed. But I have found that a rational and often successful treatment depends first upon detoxicating the patient. This is followed by the attempt to build up the asthma victim's adrenals, thus removing as much strain as possible from the congested liver. The most reliable detoxication procedure consists of physical rest for the organs involved. The patient is given a diet of natural antidotes. Many alkaline metals are needed but always in *organic* form, for the liver can never assimilate inorganic material. But it can assimilate sodium from the squash, cucumber or melon family and from papayas or yams; potassium from green leaves of vegetables; calcium from the stems of plants; vitamins and trace elements (minerals) from the juice of raw root vegetables. A soup prepared from some of these vegetables that are most easily assimilated by the patient is of utmost value dietetically.

Not a trace of salt should be allowed the asthmatic patient. Salt (sodium chloride) is frequently used to excess on foods because it stimulates the adrenal glands, but it is really a highly corrosive drug—a former embalming fluid which cannot be used in the body economy. But *organic* salt, as found in vegetables, is useful and non-toxic. It is this form of sodium chloride which is vitally necessary to the body.

If the urine is carefully examined several times a day while the patient is on a corrected diet, it will be noted that it gradually becomes lighter in color and contains less of the toxic material that characterizes the average asthmatic's urine. It is extremely important to know when the toxemia of the blood has cleared, for then real nourishment must be given, otherwise the patient may develop starvation acids and have a recurrent attack. He may also digest his own tissues, which are exceedingly toxic, thus flooding his blood with a fresh concentration of his own chief asthmatic poisons.

Nourishment for him must consist of protein. Raw or very rare beef or lamb supplies, even to children, the most necessary amino acids with the least amount of liver congestion. This food may be given as soon as breathing becomes more comfortable. The number and size of feedings depend upon the patient's ability to handle the food. After some weeks, with steady improvement and weight gain, other foods may be tried. As a rule the concentrated starches are forbidden, as are such easily putrefiable proteins as dairy products and eggs. It is finally possible for the patient to arrive at a proper combination of foods when he learns which foods are most beneficial and easily digested by him.

THE COMMON COLD

Sir William Osler once declared: "There is just one way to treat a cold, and that is with contempt." But when President Johnson caught a cold during Inauguration week, it became a front-page story, practically as important as a declaration of war. Americans in general disagree with Osler; in seeking relief from the annoying symptoms of the common cold, they spend nearly a quarter of a billion dollars a year for pills, nose drops, sprays and cough medicines. Colds justly merit the adjective "common," for they are more prevalent than all other illnesses combined.

To understand the common cold we should know that the mucous membrane or inner skin of the respiratory tract may be conveniently divided into three parts: (1) the mucous membrane of the nose and sinuses; (2) the posterior throat and nasopharynx; (3) the mucous membrane of the bronchial tree, _i.e._, the lungs. These mucous membrane areas are under the influence of the thyroid gland, as are all mucous membranes. The cold, or typical inflammation resulting in a catarrhal exudation, is caused by a vicarious elimination of toxins specifically directed by the thyroid gland.

Four different degrees of mucous-membrane inflammation are possible in the common cold, depending primarily upon the nature of the toxin eliminated. First, there is a simple redness and irritation with exudation of a clear, salty-tasting fluid; an example of this is the dripping of the nose during the early stages of a cold. Such an inflammation involves only the most superficial layers of the mucous membrane; the layer containing the mucous glands is scarcely involved, which is evident from the lack of mucus in the watery secretion of the cold's early stage. If the main irritant to be eliminated is sodium chloride, this type of cold may last only a day or two, followed by quick recovery. Dilute solutions of silver nitrate sprayed or swabbed on the membrane inactivate the irritation of the sodium chloride by changing the highly soluble sodium chloride into insoluble silver chloride. All types of catarrhal exudates contain a high concentration of sodium chloride, otherwise known as common table salt. Salt, in my opinion, is one of the condiments universally used to excess.

The second degree of inflammation is characterized by a deeper burn, which involves the serous and the upper mucous layer, includ-

ing the mucous glands. The secretions exuded contain both serous
fluid and clear mucus. As the degree of inflammation depends upon
the concentration and chemistry of the toxins eliminated, it may
be concluded that the result here would be a moderate cold lasting
three or four days.

The third degree of inflammation follows a still deeper burn,
involving the lower layer of mucous glands, with a moderate
amount of injury, including destruction of the mucous cells. Germs
gather to digest the products of the inflammation and white blood
cells rush in to destroy the germs. The secretion is now mucopuru-
lent, which means that pus is present as well as mucus and serum.
This type of cold lasts ten days or more and is severe in character.

The fourth degree of inflammation involves all the preceding
layers plus the deepest layer, which is rich in blood vessels. Blood
can be present in the exudation, which at this stage would be
termed mucopurulent-hemorrhagic. If large blood vessels are corroded by the toxins, a dangerous hemorrhage may follow. This type
of cold is exceedingly severe and may last several weeks. And even
after this cold is considered cured, several weeks or more may be
needed for complete repair of tissues.

There is really nothing mysterious in the cause of the common
cold, although it is a subject of much debate among medical men.
Colds are most prevalent in the winter months mainly because
there is much less active skin function during this time, with con-
siderably less skin respiration and perspiration. Also, the average
diet contains fewer fruits and vegetables during the winter and a
higher concentration of salt. When people are less active, they tend
to be constipated and also to overeat, especially during the holiday
season—Thanksgiving, Christmas and New Year's—with consequent impairment of the liver and kidney function and general
metabolism. A cold often follows these celebrations.

The fact that there is always a toxic state before a cold is merely
another way of saying that the concentration of poisons in the
blood has reached a level too high for the liver and kidneys to strain
out; thus the thyroid, as the third line of defense, comes into play.

If the thyroid must tackle the job, catarrhal inflammation will result. In essence, the common cold is nothing but a catarrhal inflammation.

Germs are not the cause; they are merely scavengers that eat up the toxic wastes and the dead cells following inflammation. But the danger is that waste products of the germs that have fed on the dead cells together with the irritation from the toxins themselves may be absorbed into the blood of the cold victim.

Remedies recommended for treatment of the common cold are legion; the effect of most of them is to suppress symptoms and lower the temperature. But these remedies are more harmful than helpful, because they irritate the already overworked liver, which is the detoxication center of the body. The popular antibiotics act chiefly by violently stimulating the adrenal glands; this will often clear up a toxemia, but if the adrenals are weak or depleted, the disease runs a chronic and frequently recurring course instead.

Science, for all its efforts, has not yet found a specific treatment for the common cold. Since the whole body is congested with poisons, it is advisable to remove all the strain until some degree of elimination of poisons can take place. Muscular rest is imperative; therefore, the patient should be put to bed promptly. But muscular rest is not half as important as glandular rest, since the liver is greatly overstrained and fatigued.

There are two methods of lightening the liver's burden: *The first is to stop the ingestion of proteins, sugars, starches and fats; the second is to try to find out the chemical character of the toxemia and to give frequent doses of what might be termed therapeutic antidotes.* These may be plain water, diluted fruit juices, diluted vegetable soups (without meat or other seasoning) or diluted raw vegetable juices. Sometimes cooked fruit juices, well diluted, are needed. This type of treatment is called fasting. When properly followed and combined with rest, it is the ideal procedure and promises freedom from complications.

Sir William Osler believed the cold should be treated with "contempt," but he also always followed a simple and effective prescription for the illness: bed rest, a good book to read, no food. The aphorism of Hippocrates—"If you feed a cold, you will have to starve a fever"—is as true today as when he wrote it, although it has been corrupted into "Feed a cold and starve a fever." But as long as man, steeped in superstition and fear, believes that he is the innocent victim of an outside attack, he will continue to use some form of treatment to "drive out" the cold and kill the germs.

DIABETES

Diabetes is a chronic condition in which the body cannot metabolize a part of the food eaten, notably sugars and starches. It ranks seventh in the causes of death due to disease in this country. There are about 1,800,000 diagnosed diabetics, plus possibly a million or more who do not know they have the disease. Insulin and the "anti-diabetes pills" were acclaimed "life savers" for diabetics. But are they?

At the risk of again being called "controversial," I must disagree. Insulin is a toxic substance which has a harmful effect on the blood vessels. Its continued use causes different types of arterial disease. Careful observation shows that the body can stand the poison of insulin injection for about twenty-five years at most and then the patient's arteries disintegrate and life comes to an end. In diabetics there is always a very toxic background and the thyroid gland is usually overstimulated. Insulin puts a brake on thyroid activity and thus slows up the discharge of sugar into the blood from the liver. The anti-diabetes pills also have the ability to put a brake on thyroid activity. But the pills' effect is so much weaker and their toxic effect on the other organs, especially the liver, is so much greater, that they are really more dangerous than insulin. What is accomplished with diabetic pills is not worth the risk of taking them.

In treating adult diabetics I have been able to control sugar in the urine by diet alone. (In diabetic children, where the natural prognosis is very poor even with the finest of treatment, the best I have been able to do is cut down the use of insulin from forty units a day to five or ten but not to do without it entirely.)

I place the patient on a cleaner diet. The most valuable regime for the diabetic patient is a vegetable diet—cooked, non-starchy vegetables and vegetable soups. My aim is to aid the depleted pancreas, whose chief chemical element is a potassium compound. So the potassium-rich vegetables are of special value. If the potassium level can be built up, this not only rebuilds the pancreas but neutralizes a great deal of the acidity which is always in the background in diabetes.

The best way to handle a diabetic case, I have found, is to take him off insulin and to put him to bed. If the patient will not accept this and the rather rigorous diet, then I am powerless to help. The diet consists of lightly cooked non-starchy vegetables, like celery, parsley, zucchini and string beans, liquified in a blender and used as a soup. The patient remains on this until the urine becomes sugar-free by test. He stays in bed to conserve his energy in order to give the liver and the pancreas every possible chance to do their work unmolested from the acids of exertion. It may take from one day to four days or more to get the patient sugar-free.

He is allowed then to resume his normal activities while following a fairly careful diet; he is watched to see how long it takes to develop sugar again. When this happens, he is once again "fasted" in bed on the vegetable soup. Generally then it takes half the length of time to get him sugar-free. What I work for is an ideal diet for his particular case which will maintain him sugar-free and still give him enough energy to do a certain amount of work. A serious diabetic case is always a sick patient, whether or not he is sugar-free. And he will always have a deranged pancreas and to a great extent a deranged liver, so that one can never expect him to be one-hundred-percent perfect and able to live normally. In a mild case, however, the patient will respond beautifully to a starch- and sugar-restricted diet, to losing weight if necessary and to establishing good living habits.

HAY FEVER

Hay fever develops after there is an atrophy of the nasal and sinus mucous membranes. These membranes, when catarrhal, are extremely sensitive to irritating pollens, dust, animal exhalations, smog and/or chemicals which often cause violent sneezing and coughing when they come in contact with the sensitive, inflamed membrane. But the inflammation comes first and the irritation follows. When there is no catarrhal state, there is no hay fever, no matter what irritant is inhaled.

Here again is seen the process of vicarious elimination with a definite salty background. Hay fever sufferers, with few exceptions, have overindulged in table salt. This explains the popularity of silver applications as a cure, just as silver nitrate is used as a spray or swab in the treatment of a cold. But not only is excess salt eliminated but also toxic products of starch and protein indigestion. The high vitamin content of the fresh spring and summer fruits often stimulates the endocrine glands to overactivity and produces a crisis which we call hay fever. That explains why it is so prevalent in those times of the year when the pollen count is highest. But remember that the irritants inhaled at these times do not *cause* hay fever unless the mucous membrane is already inflamed (a speck of dust or other foreign body can cause a much more violent irritation in a sore eye than in a normal eye).

Using less salt, abstaining from toxemia-producing proteins and starches, and exercising greater care in the selection and amount of fresh fruit ingested comprise the first step in controlling the toxemia that causes the disease. Nor must the endocrines be forgotten, for heat stimulates the adrenal glands. These glands, when overactive, reciprocally stimulate the thyroid gland through the sympathetic nervous system. Then the thyroid causes vicarious elimination through the mucous membranes, thus aggravating the hay fever symptoms. Therefore, hay fever sufferers often find relief in colder climates. But if the adrenals are weak and the thyroid still strong enough to cause vicarious elimination when toxemia exists, the victim will not benefit by moving to a colder climate.

WOMEN'S AILMENTS

Most women usually overlook and endure abnormal menstrual functions. Blinded by the idea that the average represents the normal, women have been led to believe that many pathological states are normal simply because they are prevalent. I believe that the woman who continually takes aspirin for her ills is really suffering from a state of toxemia. Because the liver is failing as a filter, the blood stream has become poisoned by products of indigestion which, if not eliminated through vicarious channels, may carry the person rapidly toward a terminal disease such as tuberculosis or cancer. One of the common safety valves occurs in the female. The menstrual function, instead of fulfilling its natural purposes, is turned into a sort of garbage filter, resulting in a condition of chronic inflammation of the uterus. After years of trying to help cleanse the blood of irritating toxins, the uterus becomes so tumorous or degenerated that hysterectomy offers the only solution to far too many women.

A study of the average menstrual function shows many abnormalities. Pain, cramps, excessive flow are so common that there are a host of popular patent medicines for their relief. When toxic blood seeks an outlet through the uterus via the menstrual function, the resulting inflammation and irritation to the delicate mucous membrane throw the organ into spasms which are registered as pain or cramps. If the toxin is milder or more dilute, the patient simply feels a sense of heaviness or congestion in the pelvis. Once the flow has started, nature pours out as much toxic material from the blood as possible, inflaming the deeper layers of the uterus. What should be a normal flow develops into a hemorrhage, sometimes lasting for days, reducing the patient to a constant state of anemia. Nervousness, insomnia, headache, distressing fatigue may follow. The kidneys may not be able to filter certain diffusible poisons, so that a mild-to-severe edema occurs, evidenced by an increase in body weight.

The quality of the menstrual blood varies according to the chemistry of the toxic material. Bright red, profuse, odorless blood accompanied by severe uterine cramps indicates that the preponderant irritant comes from improper digestion of sugars and starches. The offending toxins are acids which have failed to be completely oxidized to carbon dioxide and water. On the other hand, if the menstrual blood is dark, odorous, clotted and stringy, the toxins of protein indigestion or putrefaction are present. Eggs, cheese and well-cooked meat can cause most offensive odors in the menstrual blood. Thus it is obvious that under chemical duress the uterus, which nature selected as the organ of reproduction, can become an organ for the elimination of putrid waste.

Not only does the unhealthy woman endure much suffering during her menstrual years, but she faces an even more exasperating ordeal at the menopause. The "normal" menopause in the healthy woman is symptomless. The periods simply stop. That is all.

But the toxic female, who has had much relief from the burden of her poisons through menstrual channels, is faced at the menopause by one of the greatest crises of her life. It is as though a dam has suddenly obstructed a raging stream. The backwaters flood and devastate many acres of body tissues. A whole series of new ailments arise, among them: menopausal hot flashes, "nervous breakdown," headache, arthritis, neuritis, mild or severe insanity, gastric and intestinal indigestion, weakness and prostration, irritating vaginal discharge, palpitation of the heart, shortness of breath.

Unfortunately, this cessation of vicarious elimination through the uterus may bring a still more disastrous result. When the gate of exit is closed by the menopause, the toxins continue to gravitate in the direction of the uterus and infiltrate it. Gradually, inflammation increases and eventually a watery discharge, with a characteristic metallic odor, may begin to ooze from the lymphatic vessels of the womb. *This is a first warning of cancer.*

It is to be hoped there will come a time, after careful study of the patient's body chemistry, diet chemistry, glandular heredity and kidney-liver function, when the prospective cancer case can be taught to correct her chemical mistakes and thereby avoid becoming a cancer victim.

Happily, much relief can be offered to the patient suffering from milder disturbances of menstruation and menopause. I have found that the painful period may be relieved by reducing the concentration of toxins in the blood, best accomplished by limiting the diet for one or two days just before the period begins. If the appropriate antidote is an acid, diluted fruit juices should be taken every hour; if an alkali is indicated, diluted raw vegetable juice, yeast or meatless vegetable soup is the prescription. No other food should be taken for this day or two. As the blood toxemia is reduced, the urine becomes less acid and lighter in color. Therefore frequent checks of the urine are a valuable criterion to indicate the necessary duration of the limited diet. As the blood clears, the endocrine glands function more normally.

The patient suffering menopausal difficulties should try to live within certain dietary, emotional and physical limitations. By reducing the toxemia through diet and improved elimination, the most distressing symptoms can often be relieved; symptoms which, after all, only indicate that the thyroid is trying to help out in a difficult situation.

Finally, it is evident in this short summary of diseases that vicarious elimination plays a role in each ailment. The name of each particular disease is determined by which organ is involved. In every case there is some type of glandular imbalance or subnormality with a consequent attempt toward compensation by another gland. Rational therapy depends upon detoxication followed by repair and willingness on the part of the patient to reorganize his life so that he does not overstep the margin of efficiency for the particular organ involved.

PART III

FOOD
IS YOUR
BEST
MEDICINE

14

Proteins Are Body Builders

> When mighty roast beef was the Englishman's food,
> It ennobled our hearts, and enriched our blood,
> Our soldiers were brave and our courtiers were good.
> Oh! the roast beef of old England!
>
> —RICHARD LEVERIDGE (1670–1758)

Americans, even more than Britain's old Beefeaters, are very protein-conscious indeed these days, bombarded in newspapers and magazines with educational material on "essential amino acids" and "adequate versus inadequate proteins." It will, therefore, come as no surprise to anyone that in order to survive, the body needs proteins (literally, "of first importance") in its foodstuffs. We know that every living thing, from an elephant to the smallest invisible virus, is essentially protein. A wholesome diet must be rich in protein, because this valuable substance is being continually broken down for building or repair, for formation of body regulators, burned to yield energy and changed into carbohydrates and fat.

But does today's American diet, for infants through oldsters—following the popularized campaign of food promoters in the press—rely *too* heavily on protein foods? In jumping on the protein bandwagon, are we wolfing down too much meat—becoming, in fact, over-proteinized? Have recent scientific nutritional discoveries tended to overemphasize the true importance of protein in our diet? Those of us who think so call this the "protein era" (one U.S. Food and Drug Administration official, worried about the claims of the so-called high-protein breakfast cereals in advertising, laments "the miserable protein chaos"). And we believe that in the explosion engendered by this and other campaigns for protein in the diet, some vital facts have become almost buried.

Certainly, *protein, as a basic constituent of every living cell, is vitally important in our diet.* Americans do not have to search far; they find a superabundance of protein in meat, poultry, fish, eggs, milk, cheese, and such protein-rich vegetables as grain products and legumes like beans, peas and peanuts.

However, after what I show you in this and the following chapter, I think you will agree with me that while proteins are truly body builders, they may *sometimes, under certain conditions, also act as body killers.*

For an understanding of the functioning of protein within the body, we must start with the atom—the simplest chemical substance known. An *atom* is designated by one letter, for example, O for oxygen, H for hydrogen and N for nitrogen. It is possible for two atoms to combine: for example, sodium (Na) and chlorine (Cl) make common table salt. The combination of two or more atoms is called a *molecule.* As the number of atoms in the molecule becomes greater, the size of the molecule naturally increases. Simple chemical substances, such as NaCl, contain a small number of atoms and are known in chemistry as inorganic compounds. Highly complex combinations of many atoms, usually built around the carbon atom, are called organic compounds.

The organic molecules, called *colloids,* which compose the plant or animal body are highly complex. When colloid molecules contain nitrogen, they are known as protein colloids. Animal bodies and plants are composed of protein colloids. The plant digs its roots into the wet soil and absorbs the inorganic mineral elements, which are transformed by the energy of sunlight into organic colloidal substances. Along comes a steer who eats the plant; his digestive process converts the plant protein into muscle. The natural food of man is the plant or the animal which ate the plant. We know that man's body cannot grow, develop and repair damage without an adequate supply of the right kind of protein.

Proteins form the cells of the body, whether they are the calcium.

proteins of the bones, the sodium proteins of the liver, the potassium proteins in the pancreas, the phosphorus proteins in the brain and nerves, the iron and copper proteins of the red blood or the sulphur proteins of the connective tissues. Even the trace elements and the vitamins are proteins.

Man obtains his necessary proteins from either animal or vegetable sources. Dairy products, eggs and animal flesh consist of what are called animal protein; all vegetables also contain some protein, peas and beans a high proportion. Much has been made of the so-called "superiority" of animal foods over plant foods as sources of protein in human diet. Unfortunately, this has given rise to a popular misconception that man cannot obtain strength and good health by getting his protein from a diet consisting only of plant food. Yet herbivorous animals build strong muscles and bones from grass and leaves alone. The elephant lives on leaves and grows his enormous tusks from the calcium protein of the leaves. The moose and elk grow huge antlers in just a few months each year, shedding them again in the winter—the moose on a diet of water plants and green leaves, the elk on leaves, twigs and grass.

During digestion and assimilation, the human body breaks down food proteins into their constituent amino acids. And it must be remembered that an amino acid, whether plant or animal in source, is *the same amino acid*, equally useful to the body as food. Man can exist upon animal or vegetable protein or both and be in good health, *providing his liver functions normally*.

A young animal's liver functions normally on milk—the universal protein. For each species of animal, there is no substitute for mother's milk, called "the most nearly perfect food." Mother's milk contains proteins, carbohydrates, fats, several vitamins and practically all the required salts. When the animal is weaned, other forms of animal or vegetable protein take its place, the nature of the protein depending upon the environment and on whether the animal is carnivorous, herbivorous or omnivorous. Protein is the most essential element in the diet; it must be supplied in adequate amounts, especially during the active growth period of man or animal. But as old age approaches, less and less is needed.

During digestion, proteins are broken down to simple molecules, called amino acids, which are the building blocks of the body tissues. Between a hundred thousand and a million different proteins exist. Science is still trying to learn why and how a protein molecule functions—an awesome problem. We do know that protein digestion begins in the stomach and continues through the small intestine. Some of the amino acids reach the liver through the veins of the small intestine. The liver builds up essential body proteins from useful amino acids and eliminates the useless or harmful ones with the bile. In addition to taking nourishment the body cells must multiply and reproduce themselves. This brings us to one of the most miraculous functions of the amazing body cells, described in a previous chapter but of such great importance in the unmatched wonders of the human body that it bears repeating.

The multiplication of cells is dependent upon an iodine compound found in the thyroid hormone. This hormone is carried to the cells by white blood corpuscles called small lymphocytes. Reproduction and multiplication of cells is impossible in the absence of either the small lymphocytes or of the thyroid hormone. The rate of reproduction of cells varies greatly in the human body. During embryonic life it is very rapid; when the adult state is reached, the rate is retarded except during the stages of tissue repair, at which time the embryonic rate is again approximated. It is during the rapid growth of childhood and adolescence that the blood count shows an excess of small lymphocytes—called the leucocytosis of childhood—which is considered to be a normal state.

When body cells are injured or destroyed by accident or disease, a rapid repair and multiplication of cells must take place. To allow for this, the body supplies to the affected area a bath rich in small lymphocytes. This concentration of lymphocytes into injured or diseased tissues is an accepted histological fact. That the lymphocytes carry elements that are vitally necessary to support multiplication of cells seems plainly evident, because microscopic study shows that where there are no lymphocytes, there is no multiplication. The easy destruction and slow tissue repair in states of leucopenia (a condition of the blood characterized by fewer white cells than normal) seems to support this.

Since the small lymphocytes are necessary for the accomplishment of biological reproduction, it may not be too presumptuous to believe that they carry certain vital elements, some of which could be picked up on their journey through the vessels of the blood and lymph circulation. To demonstrate and support this statement, follow the course of a small lymphocyte from a lymphocyte-manufacturing center, such as the spleen, to its final destination, the growing cell. Leaving the spleen by lymphatic vessels, it permeates the area of the intestinal villi where it is enriched with amino acids fresh from the process of protein digestion. Nature then collects these food-filled lymphocytes into a large vessel, the lymphatic duct, and discharges them into the subclavian vein, located just under the collarbone. The blood in this vein is especially rich in thyroid hormone, because the thyroid gland discharges its secretions into the subclavian vein, facilitating a rapid thyroid impregnation of lymphocytes, without which growth and reproduction of body cells is impossible.

The tremendous importance of the impregnation of small lymphocytes with thyroid hormone is again suggested by the proximity of the thymus gland (another lymphocyte-manufacturing center) to the thyroid itself. Many of the thymus veins empty directly into the thyroid vein. The size and activity of the thymus during the early period of growth and adolescence, simultaneous with that physiological leucocytosis (increase in white blood cells) of childhood and its final atrophy when the body has reached maturity, would strengthen the assumption that the thymus is the chief lymphocyte-manufacturing center during early life. In order to keep the thymus and the thyroid in good functional order, the proteins of the growing child must be carefully selected. For the thyroid, the chief iodine center of the body, proteins rich in *available* iodine must be furnished; for the thymus and the lymphocytes, amino acids containing phosphorus. Supplying the right kind and correct amount of protein is, indeed, one of the most important steps in the growth and development of the individual.

One important point to remember is that because protein is a highly stimulating food and because its taste is so pleasant, it is often consumed in excess of actual body needs. "It has been aptly demonstrated," says Dr. P. H. Mitchell in *The Mitchell Textbook of General Physiology*, "that when food protein is increased, the corresponding increase in total nitrogen equilibrium lags behind. Eventually, the body exhibits nitrogen equilibrium at a new and higher level. Meanwhile, a considerable amount of new protein *must* have accumulated in the body. No compensatory excretion of an excess of nitrogen-containing waste products occurs. Correspondingly, an experimental animal that has been fed protein in excess of its actual needs may be expected to resist the effect of a protein deficient diet for a relatively long period. The *organs* that serve as limited accumulators of protein include the liver, the intestinal tissue and the kidneys. They are known to increase in weight and in their protein content in an experimental animal after it has been fed on a high protein diet."

Recent statistics show that the average American male (heaviest meat eater in the world) eats his weight in meat each year, approximately 172 pounds of it. It is the nutritional fashion, these days, to prescribe meat up to three times a day for adults and growing children. Meat is intensely satisfying to the taste; it has a warming effect on the body. After protein food is consumed, its metabolism-stimulating effect persists for many hours. That is why the sensation of hunger is slow to return after a steak is eaten.

Because of its stimulating effect, too much protein in the diet often gives a sense of well-being, but there is, to the informed physician, a great difference between health and this type of stimulation. Few people, and too often not even members of the medical profession, recognize the difference between health and stimulation or the fact that stimulation may lead to degenerative disease. When this happens, it may be necessary that a protein-free diet (as far as is possible) be maintained for several years in order to allow the individual to use up his protein excess and so finally to return to a normal nitrogen balance.

When this excess has resulted from *the overeating of natural* foods (*that is, foods as found in nature rather than foods refined by man, such as white sugar and flour, etc.*) *properly prepared and well handled by the liver, the outcome may not be particularly harmful.* This is an important point to consider. Natural foods properly prepared does not mean a dinner of fried, pickled, preserved, brined or smoked meat or fish topped off with apple pie. If you eat improperly, a good part of your body's activity consists of just getting rid of the "non-food" you have fed it. When improper, overcooked proteins are eaten—those which putrefy in the intestine and acidify the liver—a foundation is laid for degenerative disease. This can only end disastrously.

Since the liver is the largest and most important organ in the body, let us look at its evolution to see what kind of protein it is best equipped to handle. We are told that the "animal age" covered a period of about sixty million years, and the age of man's development about a million years. Man's liver evolved from the animal's liver. The diet of primitive man was exceedingly simple. For many thousands of years food was eaten entirely uncooked. In cases of severe debilitated states of health and terminal disease, ancient peoples, as well as present-day primitive tribes, recognized the value of a raw protein diet. Hippocrates prescribed milk for tuberculosis and later physicians used fresh raw blood as a beneficial treatment of this disease.

Not only raw blood but raw eggs have long been of therapeutic value in the diet. To insure a state of health and strength during ordeals, the Indians of northern Canada consumed the raw adrenal glands of animals. Raw liver was commonly used by the Plains Indians to rehabilitate exhausted and diseased people. Those in excellent health also regularly included raw liver in their diet. Even today raw fish is used by the Eskimos as well as by the South Sea Islanders for the cure of disease. And the final reversion, in the debility of old age, to a raw-milk diet proved the adequacy of the simple raw-protein diet. For all the wrong reasons, the press, some years ago, made much of the fact that John D. Rockefeller, Sr., in his last years, subsisted on a diet composed entirely of raw human milk, supplied by a group of wet nurses.

Milk is most easily digested in the raw state. High-protein vegetables, such as the legumes, seeds and grains, have some degree of value, but are all digested with more difficulty than animal protein and the late aftereffects may be harmful. But in the final analysis, the choice of protein—even of good protein—depends upon the individual liver metabolism.

Finally, let me emphasize the importance of supplying the right kind and amount of protein, especially for the growing child. True, proteins are body builders, but only the *right kind* of proteins which the human liver can handle will build the right kind of bodies. Remember that we still have the cave man's liver and must select and use our proteins with discrimination. Because the sheep still lives a natural life in hill and mountain pastures, its meat is the most valuable meat for human consumption. *But it must be eaten rare.* Beef is next best. Fish, fowl and sea foods, unless eaten raw, are usually overcooked, therefore likely to putrefy in the intestines. The same applies to pork (although I never prescribe it), glandular organs, tripe and brains. Eggs are valuable for the yolk, which is best eaten raw or lightly cooked; the egg white should never be cooked.

Depleted adrenal glands, for example, can often be rapidly rebuilt by the ingestion of raw egg yolks, which are rich in lecithin, a phospholypoid. The yolks supply the needed phosphorus.

I had occasion to use this therapy to rehabilitate a famous Hollywood columnist. One day while she was out walking, she fainted. When she came into my office she was frightened, for she is the kind of woman who prides herself on being able to take care of herself at all times. She had been working terribly hard, she told me, had recently completed a book, made all sorts of personal appearances, including a lecture tour through Canada, and on top of this she was writing seven columns a week and two magazine stories a month. My examination showed what must be obvious from the foregoing: she was totally exhausted. I insisted that she place herself in my care immediately.

"Why?" she asked me. "Just because I'm tired?"

"No," I told her truthfully, "but because if you ever come close to being this tired again, the next time you faint you may not get up."

I put her in a dimly lit room, forbade her to talk with anyone or watch television, and placed her on a diet of softly cooked egg yolks, and soup made from string beans and zucchini.

"I'll go out of my mind," she said.

"We'll see," I answered.

The first day she tossed and turned and slept fitfully. The following day she slept for five hours straight, the next for ten hours. After that it kept increasing until she was sleeping fourteen hours daily and relaxing for the remainder. At the end of ten days I told her she could get up and go back to work, "if you take it easy."

She has been well ever since.

15

Proteins Can Be Body Killers

> His food
> Was glory, which was poison to his
> mind
> And peril to his body.
> —SIR HENRY TAYLOR (1800–1886)

If we were to change the word "glory" to "an overabundance of proteins" in the above poem, it would ruin a beautiful metaphor, but it would be a correct assumption from the standpoint of nutrition and disease.

Proteins can be body killers, if we are not watchful of our diet.

Protein foodstuffs are indispensable to the living organism, for they are basic constituents of every living cell, whether it is muscle, brain or fingernails of humans, or wood and leaves of trees, fur of animals or any vegetable that grows.

Protein can be burned in the human body to make calories in the same way that fat can and it can also be converted into carbohydrates by the body. But neither carbohydrates nor fats can act as substitutes for protein. Actually, then, it is impossible for the body to grow and thrive and repair damage without an adequate supply of the proper kind and quantity of protein. For each animal and plant, the type of protein required differs somewhat. So, in trying to discover which type of protein is best suited to the human body, we must first ask ourselves just what protein actually does, in and for that human body.

To illustrate, let us again view the body as a gasoline engine. The energy and heat of the engine are derived from the combustion of gasoline, which is rich in carbon. In the body energy and heat come from the proper oxidation of sugars, in which carbon predominates. Sugar comes either directly from sugar ingested or from sugar derived from the breaking down of starches and fats. The gasoline engine is built of metals; when worn, it must be repaired with new parts consisting of the same materials. Similarly, the body is built of proteins; it must be repaired with proteins. Gasoline must be stored in accessory tanks until needed, which makes the whole engine structure more bulky. *Excess sugars, starches and fats create the same effect in the body.* If too much metal is added to the gasoline engine, such as extra carburetors, piston rings, cylinders, etc., the engine becomes cluttered and crowded and, as a result, it runs poorly or breaks down completely. *Excessive proteins in the human body can also make it run poorly or break down completely.*

Until comparatively recently the medical profession believed that excess protein was always eliminated, chiefly by the kidneys. Now we know that excess protein can be stored up in the body cells with disastrous results. For example, *one of the main sources of so-called "over-acidity" is excess protein in the tissues.* This will come as news to most people. But the truth is that the body becomes so saturated with extra proteins that nitrogen metabolism is disturbed. All proteins are composed of smaller units called amino acids, the true building stones, which make new tissue and maintain existing tissue. But the presence of too many amino acids upsets the acid-base equilibrium of the body. Disastrous consequences follow.

Many medical men are seriously concerned over what they call the "protein mania" in food manufacturers' advertising. I agree completely with one of them, the eminent pediatrician, Dr. L. Emmett Holt, Jr., who wrote in *Postgraduate Medicine:*

In light of our present uncertainties and the suggestive evidence that we may have passed the optimum protein intake for meeting some of our important stresses, are we justified in continuing to enrich our diets with protein? The pressures to do so are great. The cereal industry has become protein-conscious and has begun to reinforce its products with protein and amino acids. Protein content and protein quality have become sales gimmicks in the food industry. As doctors we want to play it safe and to subject our patients to the least possible risk. But is it playing it safe to go along with this trend, or is it time we called a halt until we can evaluate what our present diets are doing before we go further along the road of protein 'enrichment'?

Much can be learned from the wisdom of nature as to the body's actual protein requirements. One simple example of these is the need for milk in the unique pattern of growth of various species of young animals. The calf grows rapidly, doubling the weight of its bones every month, on milk containing an ample supply of calcium-protein and albumen-protein (muscle-producing) supplied by the mother cow. The goat grows more slowly, therefore needs less of similar proteins in its milk. But the human baby grows still more slowly. On ample mother's milk, the newborn baby doubles its weight during the first six months of its life. Never again will it repeat that performance in any six months, yet the mother's milk contains the lowest *protein ratio of any mammal.* And when maturity is reached and the growing process is slowed down, a minimum amount of protein is needed—just enough to maintain what is called "nitrogen equilibrium." Then, as old age advances, even this minimum becomes less and less. It is true, however, that after injury, surgery or great physical exhaustion, temporary increase is required.

Unhappily, the stimulation resulting from too much protein in the diet, especially meat (muscle tissue), is often mistaken for health. And it follows that this has given rise to the mistaken belief that a "high-protein diet" is always beneficial and greatly to be desired, especially when the idea is encouraged by those with protein to sell through expensive advertising. Tiny jars of baby foods containing meat products fill the grocery shelves. Mothers, seeking only what is best for baby according to the advertisements, fill their carts with a vast assortment. *But nature says that milk is the required food for the growing infant; in fact, it is the only food made specifically for it.*

Cats, of course, are essentially carnivorous animals; still, very young kittens develop convulsions when put on a meat diet in laboratory experiments. These convulsions are the direct result of a toxemia originating from the indigestion of improper proteins. The kitten's liver is not yet able to metabolize this kind of protein. It is my belief that the increase of certain kinds of serious diseases in children, such as rheumatic heart disease, leukemia and polio, seems to suggest a possible origin of improper proteins in the diet. Also, the incidence of cancer and heart disease in middle age has more than doubled during the last several decades, perhaps pointing to the same kind of dietetic errors. When I first began to practice, I would see two or three cases of cancer a year. Nowadays, I see six to eight a month. Can the over-protein craze of the last twenty-five years, started by propaganda of the meat packers, be the cause of the increase of cancer?

If we wish to learn more about what happens to the protein that we eat, it is necessary to turn our attention to the chemistry of the liver. Even if it may bore you, I repeat: man has come through the evolution of the last million years with practically the same liver with which he started. His liver is "styled" for certain kinds of protein, in quality and quantity; health and longevity necessarily depend upon supplying that type of protein in the diet.

We know from the study of primitive man, as exemplified by several tribes existing at present in the Australian bush, that the early dietary protein consisted of raw protein. Meat, blood and marrow were used in their raw state. We know, too, that Eskimos and Indians of the Pacific Northwest ate raw fish and raw whale meat. Today, the Eskimo boils some of his meat, but usually only to thaw it. We have scientific proof that the Eskimos, although restricted by the confinement of sub-freezing temperatures, represented one of the finest physical types to be found anywhere—with sound bones and teeth—*before* they succumbed to the civilized diet of the white man.

Explorer Vilhjalmur Stefansson's experiments on diet in the Arctic provided much valuable information concerning protein digestion. Stefansson, who lived for years in the Arctic on nothing but meat and fat, soon found that travel there was impeded by the transportation of bulky provisions. Why not, he reasoned, capture food en route, especially during the long winter, when the tundra was frozen solid? Seal was plentiful and could be captured at the breathing holes in the ice. An occasional polar bear wandered into camp, and bear, he found, was good to eat.

He had previously learned from the Eskimos that their good health depended upon a raw meat diet, including blood, liver and bone marrow, mainly from seal, walrus and fish. At one time he took a group of robust young men, mostly college students, into the Arctic, provided them with a raw-meat diet, upon which they remained strong, warm and in good physical condition during the entire trip. At first the young men found the raw-meat diet nauseating and foreign to their taste; during early weeks they often vomited the food. But eventually they became accustomed to it and ate with gusto, suffering neither indigestion nor constipation. They discovered, however, that cooking or adding salt to their meat caused violent indigestion. Stefansson repeated this dietary experiment several times. And Donald MacMillan, another Arctic explorer, also demonstrated the value of Stefansson's diet.

Raw meat is the most practical food in the Far North, not only because it is the only available food but also because it is both heating and stimulating in that climate. In the tropics, though, such a diet would be disastrous. Wise nature has offered man a variety of fresh fruit instead.

One of the questions presented by Stefansson's experiment was: Why do cooked meats cause indigestion, and, if persisted in, disease? For an answer, the chemistry of the urine was studied. It was demonstrated that when meat was eaten in its natural, raw state, the urine did not contain the putrefactive acids of protein indigestion. This led to the observation and conclusion that the more protein was cooked, the greater was the amount of putrefactive products in the urine and even in the sweat and other body secretions. The colloid chemistry term for raw protein is *hydrophile colloid*. Cooked protein is a *hydrophobe colloid*. This means simply that the molecules are arranged differently; in the hydrophobe colloid, into a form not so easily assimilated by the human digestive organs. A simple example is the difference between raw egg white and hard-boiled egg white. The first is soluble in water, non-putrefactive in the intestines and behaves in a special way toward acids, bases and salts. Many major and minor maladies arise from the toxemia that follows the ingestion of cooked proteins.

The results of these experiments, although convincing, were never given much prominence. (At this point I would like to make it clear that I do not eat raw meat or any meat, for that matter, because I do not digest it well. Nor do I prescribe raw meat for my patients even though it is healthier, except in extreme instances where it is tolerated and only if they like it better that way.) But rare or underdone meat is appealing to some people's taste and is more acceptable to the liver. I have found in my practice that the amount of putrefactive acids resulting from eating lightly cooked meats can easily be neutralized by generous amounts of raw and cooked non-starchy vegetables eaten at the same meal. When the "well-done steak and French-fried potato man" among my patients switches to rare lamb chops, steamed zucchini, potato and a big green salad, he is rewarded by an improvement in health. Happily, raw milk and raw eggs present no taste problems to most patients.

The monumental work of the late Francis F. Pottenger, Jr., has proved beyond question the unhealthy nature of cooked animal protein. Dr. Pottenger experimented with cats, which are naturally carnivorous animals. They remained in excellent health on a diet of raw protein alone. Over a period of five years, using 109 cats, he made some convincing and irrefutable observations. All feeding was supervised by him and all experiments were carefully controlled. No cats in the entire experiment—often siblings of the same litter—developed disease as long as they remained on a raw-protein diet. In fact, they lived to a ripe old age.

But the cats on cooked protein all became sick and developed diseases similar to those seen in man: pyorrhea and loss of teeth, loss of hair, rarefaction of bones, arthritis, gastritis, atrophy and cirrhosis of the liver; degenerative processes in the brain and spinal cord were commonly observed. Dr. Pottenger's work represents a brave step in the right direction, but the opposition has been strong. Not only is the eating of cooked animal protein a stimulating habit of historical duration, but it is also the cornerstone of an entrenched and tremendously important industry. It is only to be expected that Dr. Pottenger's theories have gathered dust in the medical archives, but there are a few unorthodox practitioners (of which I am proud to be one) who do not mind espousing an unpopular cause.

Dr. Pottenger's work covers such a large field that it can only be touched on here. Those interested must study his scientific papers. Four of his observations stand out as milestones along the way toward truth:

(1) cats on a raw-protein diet remain healthy, while cats on cooked protein develop disease and die early;

(2) a cat once injured by a heated-protein diet can never entirely regain good health, no matter how carefully placed on a raw-protein diet;

(3) the liver impairment on the cooked protein diet is progressive, the bile becoming eventually so toxic in the stools that even noxious weeds refuse to grow in soil that has been fertilized by the cat's excretions;

(4) The first generation of kittens from these cats is markedly abnormal; the second is often born dead or diseased; there is no third generation as the mothers have become sterile.

The cooked proteins used in Dr. Pottenger's experiments included milk that had been pasteurized, Vitamin-D-irradiated and boiled, buttermilk, cheese and ice cream, also canned and dried milk, cooked eggs, fried, boiled or roasted meats, also salted and heat-dried meats. Dr. Pottenger's experiments were repeated by himself and verified by other scientists. The results are so convincingly evident that there is little room for doubt of their accuracy.

What happens to protein during digestion? When any one kind of protein is eaten, the liver automatically prepares to digest it. This function is under the control of the sympathetic nervous system and emanates from the solar plexus, a network of nerves situated at the upper end of the abdomen. The liver sets up a chemical table, let us say for protein A. But at the same meal, perhaps, protein B is eaten. As a simple example, protein A is meat and protein B is cheese. The chemical table for protein A is different from that of protein B. The liver, however, is incapable of handling the digestion of both proteins at the same time. So the solar plexus, or abdominal brain, gets busy and chooses one of three defense mechanisms to save the liver from embarrassment: (1) the meal may be vomited; this is a strong reflex in children and explains why little Johnny is so likely to throw up after a bountiful picnic of cheeseburgers, ice cream, cake, Coke and candy; (2) the muscular control of the stomach may allow one protein to pass into the small intestine while it retards the second; this amazing phenomenon has actually been shown to exist and has been proved by fractional lavage and also by X-ray evidence; (3) an increased peristalsis may result, evidenced by diarrhea.

Theologians make much of the still, small voice of the conscience. I would like to call attention to the still, small voice of the solar plexus—a part of the body to which most people pay no attention. When one eats too much food or an incompatible combination of foods, nature flashes a distress signal in the form of a belch. Most people consider a belch a digestive faux pas, but in reality it is the vestigial remains of the infant's "spitting up." Learn to heed this little warning of nature.

Acids and other waste products of protein indigestion and putrefaction are easily identified in the urine. Scientifically, they belong to the group of phenols, skatols, indoxyl-sulphuric acids, uric acid and toxic amines. Often, they are eliminated vicariously through the mucous membranes or by diffusion into the spinal fluid.

Is ice cream your best-loved dessert?

Then listen to scientific opinion concerning this bland concoction. One of the common sources of the diffusible toxin is ice cream

—that seemingly innocent and popular dessert—which is a highly putrefactive protein mixture, whether it be the best "homemade" or the crude commercial type, rich in emulsifiers. Our country consumes more ice cream than any other nation. Dr. Axel Emil Gibson, a pioneer in the study of protein putrefaction, made some interesting observations concerning the country's favorite snack in _Diet, What It Is and What It Isn't_:

> The freezing process, however, gives to the cream its last and finishing touch of physiological corruption. Quickly fermenting substances like milk, cream, fruit, etc., break down structurally at the first touch of frost. And, as the arrest of bacterial activities caused by the frost is only temporary while the molecular derangement of the frozen substance remains a permanent menace, it follows that a renewal and increase of the destructive work of the invading microbes immediately takes place when the ice cream reaches its melting point in the stomach. Hence in being able to offer physiological resistance to the microbic attack, the system is rendered helplessly negative, and like the melting glaciers of the past, which in releasing from their frigid storages the long preserved tissues of animal life, surrenders them to elemental dissolution and decay—so the ice cream, melting in the body of the individual, sets free the carcasses of the ice cream and milk cells, to lay them open to the resistless attacks of swarming and festering bacteria—though the evidence of the ghostly carnival of putrefaction escapes the taste by being masked into unrecognizability by the great deceiver—sugar. For in this physiological interment of the ice cream, the ice holds the function of the embalmer, and the sugar, the embalming fluid.

Other putrefiable products can cause the same kind of toxemia, but during the summer months there is a tremendous amount of ice cream eaten, especially by children who, hot dime in little fist, rush out to the musical vendor wagons that pass up and down the street several times a day. Is there a relationship in the fact that it is just at the peak of the ice cream season, usually July and August, that the polio epidemic strikes? Some medical men think so. And we advise parents to prohibit ice cream for their youngsters at this time.

We make this suggestion because the diffusible putrefactive acids from ice cream indigestion, when not eliminated entirely by the liver and kidneys, emerge vicariously through the mucous membranes of the nose and sinuses. These symptoms often suggest a summer cold. The polio virus feeds upon this excretion and, in the vast majority of children, causes an inflammation attended by mild fever, malaise and perhaps slight stiffness of the neck. In a few days, most children recover. If the child is extremely toxic, with subnormal adrenal glands, the virus invades the mucous membranes of the sinuses. As the membranes of the brain are in close approximation, it is a simple matter for the polio virus to spread to the brain and thence to the spinal cord, where the lesion, which results in motor paralysis, appears. Only the most toxic children are paralyzed —about 3 percent of those infected with the virus. The rarity of polio, for it is really a rare disease, is due to the small percentage of the susceptibles. These individuals usually have weak adrenal glands and a concomitant low resistance to disease, and have been heavy ice cream eaters as well as victims of other dietetic mistakes.

Many scientists have suspected a dietetic error as the cause of polio. Dr. Benjamin F. Sandler tried an experiment in Asheville, North Carolina. During one summer, the children ate no sweets whatsoever. In previous years, a large number of polio cases had occurred during the summer season. But, during the summer of Dr. Sandler's experiment, significantly enough, there were 90 percent fewer cases. Naturally, avoiding all sweets included avoiding ice cream. But if other kinds of sweet food were as dangerous, surely epidemics of polio would follow Christmas and Easter. As we know, this is not what happens. Inevitably, the finger of suspicion points strongly toward the villain—ice cream.

One would think that following this demonstration in Asheville, the city fathers would take steps to repeat the experiment. They did not. Newspapers and radio stations in North Carolina and nearby states carried Dr. Sandler's findings that in 1948, the year before the experiment, there had been 2,498 cases of polio in Asheville and only 299 reported cases in 1949, yet nothing further was done. The reason for the inaction is open to conjecture, but it goes without saying that such publicity would have endangered the sale of ice cream and other milk products in the area.

To remove such a favorite as ice cream from the diet may be considered by some as too much austerity. Dairy products in general are linked to human beings by what has been aptly called the "memory of the cells."

If adults and children, particularly, insist on eating ice cream, they should be given a mixture of fresh whipped cream, sugar and crushed fruit. Mothers find this simple to prepare as it is merely chilled in the refrigerator, not frozen. One further warning: it should never be eaten with meals or as a dessert, but either as a meal or between-meal snack, since the combination is overtaxing to the liver, especially when mixed with other animal protein or vegetable foods.

It is worth repeating again and again that *the more protein is heated or cooked,* the more its colloid form is changed. Hydrophilic colloids are converted into hydrophobic colloids. Man's primitive jungle liver is equipped to handle hydrophilic colloids, the waste products of which are easily neutralized by the liver's storehouse of sodium and eliminated in the bile as harmless complex-sodium cholates. The kidneys also assist in removing the nitrogen wastes as urea.

Structurally, the proteins differ from the sugars, starches and fats in that their composition contains nitrogen, sulphur, phosphorus, iron and many other trace elements. The sugars, starches and fats (carbohydrates and hydrocarbons) contain carbon, hydrogen and oxygen, all of which are not materially changed or damaged by heating. But the heating does alter the proteins, which then easily putrefy in the intestines and give rise to grave disturbances. This is the factor which leads to disease in both childhood and the later years.

After observing the diet of infants and young children, many medical men today marvel at the stamina of the body which withstands the often appalling diet of the first years of life. One need only compare the difference in the chemistry of the baby on an unnatural factory-concocted milk substitute and the normal breast-fed baby. In this connection, it was the venerable Oliver Wendell Holmes who observed that "a pair of substantial mammary glands has the advantage over the two hemispheres of the most learned Professor's brain, in the art of compounding a nutritious fluid for infants."

The stools of an infant on breast milk are comparatively odorless, non-irritating and soft. The baby's breath is sweet and there is no foul odor in the perspiration. Neither does the urine scald the baby's tender skin or bear a strong, offensive smell. This is because nature has provided baby with an intestinal tract suited to human milk—the specific food it was designed to utilize.

It is well-known that the mildest of all treated milks for bottle-feeding to infants is the one that has been subjected to the pasteurization process. Still, the infant's secretions, after ingestion of pasteurized milk, become odorous and irritating. Constipation often results. If the baby's urine is examined, the waste products of protein putrefaction are found. In my own practice over fifty years, I have found this repeatedly true. Commercially modified milk and baby foods are all foreign to the baby's liver digestion and may produce diarrhea, milk allergies and constipation. To overcome the latter, manufacturers sweeten their products with unnatural, artificial sugars, which increase acidity and fermentation, produce gaseous colic and toxic urine.

Milk is one of the most unstable, thermolabile of all the natural foods. Even refrigeration for twenty-four hours will rob it of some of its vitamin content and its organic structure. Pasteurization disintegrates it still more, while boiling reduces it to a useless, putrefiable mess that is tolerated by the liver with great difficulty. We can almost hear that long-suffering gland cry "Oh, no!" when confronted with a shower of hot milk.

Why do many babies apparently thrive on unnatural baby food? Because their livers are strong and their adrenals adequate; but later, from the age of three to six, we get the chronic sniffles, frequent colds, tonsillitis and croups that are found so regularly in the kinder-garten and early school years.

Those of Dr. Pottenger's cats who were fed a diet consisting solely of pasteurized milk died after three months, while the control cats, fed raw milk, remained healthy. Calves seldom live over two months on the same diet. Despite the reverence for Pasteur, en-lightened pediatricians know that pasteurization of cow's milk for infant feeding is a definitely harmful process. The large dairy in-terests use pasteurization to insure preservation, to keep milk from souring quickly. Very little milk would ever reach the large, con-gested cities if it was not pasteurized. But cleanly handled milk need not be pasteurized, as is proved by the excellent quality and sweetness of certified raw milk. When available, it should always be used.

Earlier in this chapter I mentioned that heating or cooking egg white renders it toxic. The yolk, however, is somewhat more stable, but even it is more nutritious when eaten raw or softly cooked. Meat (muscle) is best eaten raw, in which state it is sweet-tasting and easily digested; when cooked, it should be lightly broiled and rare. Lamb and beef, in that order, are the best animal proteins. It must be remembered, though, that all well-cooked proteins are digested with difficulty and produce toxemia; especially pork, veal, fish, fowl, small game, sea foods and cheeses.

Many people eat a great deal of meat and cheese and apparently remain in good health, but sooner or later nature exacts its price. It is well established that to neutralize the putrefaction products of well-cooked-protein indigestion, the liver is robbed of its sodium faster than it can be replenished by the diet, which in cooked-meat eaters is notoriously lacking in sodium-containing foods. As the liver fails, the toxemia increases.

When the adrenal glands are strong, they try to compensate for the liver's failure by superoxidation; this gives rise to increased kidney function. When both the liver and kidneys become ex-hausted, the toxemia climbs to a higher level and often necessitates an attempt at vicarious elimination through organs that normally secrete proteins. The breasts attempt to secrete toxic protein acids in the form of a poisonous milk; the uterus has an irritating secretion instead of the normal menstrual proteins. Cancer may result when the destructive qualities of acids thus vicariously eliminated rise to peak concentration. Can this be the reason why cancer in the female is so frequent in the breast and uterus?

In summing up the role of proteins as body killers, it is necessary to emphasize that natural protein for the growing animal or human baby is fresh raw milk, from nipple to mouth when possible, and that no amount of processing or additives can ever approximate or act as a substitute for natural clean raw milk. In addition, the following conclusions must be stressed: First, protein foods are the natural building blocks of the body; second, even in their most perfect state, proteins, when eaten to excess, are apt to cause an upset in body chemistry; third, several proteins at one meal are incompatible, therefore it is better to eat one protein at a time; fourth, cooking or heating animal protein renders it less digestible and increases its putrefaction during digestion.

Back in the sixteenth century, Cervantes asked, rather plaintively, in *Don Quixote:* "Can we ever have too much of a good thing?" Yes, we can—when that "good thing" is protein!

16

Vegetables as Do-It-Yourself
Therapy

> There are no more important ingredients of a properly
> constituted diet than fruits and vegetables, for they
> contain vitamins of every class, recognized and un-
> recognized.
>
> —SIR ROBERT MCCARRISON

In movies with war themes, it is frequently the Marines who come
to the rescue; in disease, it is just as frequently fresh and cooked
vegetables which do the same thing. There is usually no need to
rely on drugs. It must be remembered that all drugs are chemicals;
the same chemicals *in organic form* are found in vegetables and
other foodstuffs.

But sometimes vegetables are not easy to come by.

I am reminded of a case I once had in Idaho. I traveled across the
sagebrush for nearly a hundred miles to see a farmer who had suffered a discharging leg ulcer for several years. The whole right leg
was greatly swollen and a foul crater was located just above the
ankle.

One of the chief chemical elements I had to get into him—and
do it speedily in view of his serious condition—was alkaline vegetable juices of various types. But it was late fall and no vegetables
were growing. Nor were there any supermarkets with daily supplies

of fresh vegetables from distant farms. The only medically useful plant growing on the farm at that time of year was alfalfa.

"We'll feed him alfalfa," I said. His wife looked flabbergasted, but I managed to convince them. I instructed her to gather the tender little alfalfa shoots, mince them very fine and mix them with water and grapefruit juice, which was available at a grocery many miles away. In addition the patient was given canned vegetables, whole wheat bread and raw milk in the proper proportions. In time, adhering strictly to this regimen, the ulcer healed entirely and the swelling disappeared. Needless to say, he never resumed his diet of hog fat, white flour and white sugar.

Truly the vegetable kingdom contains our best medicines. Nevertheless, the meat-and-potatoes man looks with suspicion on any vegetable except his familiar and beloved potato. But even it was reluctantly accepted as food when first introduced in Europe in 1584. Although crop failures meant mass starvation, the peasants of Europe refused to eat the potato because they believed it caused diarrhea, poisoned the soil and helped spread the Plague. The same thing happened to the tomato when Europeans first made its acquaintance. Although the early Aztecs of Mexico considered the tomato a real "health" food and reverently offered it to their gods of healing, Europeans shunned it as the poisonous "love apple." Only sorcerers found it useful.

"And from fruits hold thyn abstinence," warned the fourteenth-century author of *Gouernayle of Helthe* when he observed that diarrheas and unpleasant symptoms increased during the fruit-ripening season. He could not know that gastrointestinal ailments came not from vegetables and fruits but from the bacteria-laden waters of the hot-weather season.

In antiquity and during the Middle Ages vegetables were held in low esteem because they didn't "stick to the ribs" as meat and cereal foodstuffs did. Even today many housewives pass up vegetables and fruits because, for the same sum, they can purchase twenty times as many calories in the cereal family, unmindful of the importance of mere traces of essential mineral elements and vitamins in vegetables.

One of the handsome sights in a supermarket is the display, like a giant Persian carpet, of many-colored vegetables and fruits. They are not only beautiful to look at but filled with healthful properties, chief of which are their natural vitamins and trace elements. *But only if they are used.* Did you know that a stalk of celery or a serving of fresh salad greens has more vitamins and minerals than a box of synthetic vitamin tablets? Unfortunately, many of us grew up in places where only potatoes and a few cold-weather vegetables were available nine months of the year, so our taste buds never knew scores of vegetables as children and we refuse to make their acquaintance as adults. Men, especially, are rigid in this regard, generally refuse all but potatoes, peas and string beans.

"Kale cost me my first husband," a woman remarked. "I hope my second will eat it."

And if he won't, you have dozens of others with which to tempt him. The vegetable kingdom differs from the animal in that it collects nourishment from the inorganic constituents of the soil. In the presence of water the roots of the plant are able to absorb mineral elements found in the earth and circulate them to the leaves, where the energy of sunlight transforms them into organic compounds containing nourishment and energy for man. Professor Albert V. Szent-Györgyi describes this process perfectly in his lecture, "Principles of Biological Oxidation":

Whatever a cell does has to be paid for—and currency of living systems, with which the cell has to pay, is energy. If there is no free energy there is no life. The sole and ultimate source of this energy is the radiation of the sun. This, however, cannot be utilized as such to maintain life, for life would fail at night if this were the case. Therefore, the radiant energy is packed into small parcels by the chloroplasts of the chlorophyll-containing plants. If the cell needs energy, it does not use radiation but unpacks those parcels of energy, called "foodstuff molecules." The two fundamental reactions of life are: (1) the making of these packages, and (2) their unpacking.

$$\text{Energy} + nCO_2 + nH_2O = nO_2 + CnH_2nOn \ldots (1)$$
$$C_nH_2O_n + nO_2 = nH_2O + nCO_2 + \text{Energy} \ldots (2)$$

(the small preceding n denotes any number of ions). Reaction (2) is the opposite of reaction (1). The first of the two reactions is performed only by the chlorophyll-containing plant cells, while reaction (2) is performed by all cells, whether of the plant itself, or of the animal which eats the plant (herbivora) or of the animal which eats the animal which ate the plant (carnivora).

It is apparent that energy is life itself and that for man, who is a mammal, the vegetable and animal kingdoms are the source—the only source—of life and energy. It must be remembered that the animal eats the vegetable or eats the animal that ate the vegetable. But man cannot eat *all* of the plants and vegetables which carpet the earth. Some are beneficial and nourishing and energizing, while others are indigestible and some are even poisonous; a number are stimulating to the body, while others are relaxing. But man, whose body is composed of the mineral elements of the earth, must seek his nourishment—his life and energy—from these same elements transformed by water and sunlight into plants.

Vegetables may be classified as starchy, non-starchy, leafy, chlorophyll-bearing, sweet, sour, semi-solid, semi-liquid. Some grow above and some below the ground; they may be any part of a plant—bulb, tuber, root, stem, seed, seed pod, leaf, fruit or blossom. Some are fatty, some non-fatty. All contain vitamins and minerals in more or less concentrated form.

The starchy vegetables include grains or other seeds, roots and tubers; the non-starchy are the leafy vegetables with their stalks and stems. Chlorophyll vegetables have the characteristic green color and are most often leafy. Sweet vegetables, such as the carrot or sweet potato, contain sugar in different forms. The characteristic tastes come from acids, such as malic, citric, oxalic and others. Vegetables are classified as semi-solid or semi-liquid according to their water content. Fats and oils are found in seeds and fruits, although traces may be found in leaves and stalks as well. Some plants are very rich in vitamin content, while others contain none beneficial to man.

When Hippocrates formulated the maxim, "Thy food shall be thy remedy," he certainly must have had in mind the medicinal qualities of vegetables. Experience has taught us that when man becomes burdened with diseases due to acid intoxication, usually from overindulgence of sweets, starches and proteins, he must turn to the alkaline vegetables for neutralization.

Dietetic histories point out that for hundreds of years, the Italians used zucchini as a cure-all. Why would they select the simple, bland vegetable for this purpose? Perhaps it was only accident, or superstition, or perhaps they found that besides being nourishing it grew well in the soil. It's more likely, however, that they reached their conclusions by trial and error, not knowing that the zucchini is an especially sodium-rich vegetable, as are other members of the squash-cucumber-melon family. *The organic sodium in zucchini, as well as in summer and crook-neck squash, is the most ideal source of refurbishing a sodium-exhausted liver.*

Such potassium-rich vegetables as string beans and the leafy plants supply the alkaline needs of the pancreas and salivary glands, which are the body's potassium storehouse. Calcium, the element necessary for the framework and support of both animals (bones) and vegetables (stalks), is to be found in the twigs and stems and supporting roots. Sodium, potassium and calcium, which the plant obtains from what is called the alkaline earths, are the three elements the body needs in greatest amount. Many other elements contained in plants are vitally necessary for the animal and human body, but in smaller doses. These are called trace elements, originating mostly in the metallic branch of the mineral kingdom; it is from this group that we receive our vitamins.

Through the ages different recipes of cooked vegetables and vegetable soups and broths have been used therapeutically. History mentions the soup of Hippocrates, the "ambrosias" of Ambroise Paré, the "composition" of Brigham Young. Today the popular vegetable combination sold in health food stores is called "potassium broth." In certain acid intoxications, manifested in diseases like neuritis, some forms of arthritis, hepatitis, nephrosis, migraine, epilepsy and cancer, the natural antidotes come from the vegetable kingdom. When a toxemia is present without symptoms of a specific disease but with liver impairment, a short fast on vegetable broth or soup is a natural and efficient treatment that will relieve the liver of its congestion and restore it to normal function.

I have found, for example, that the most valuable regimen for the diabetic patient is a short fast on non-starchy, potassium-rich vegetable broths. The diabetic's pancreas has lost its power to control the blood-sugar level. Since the pancreas' chief chemical element is potassium, the potassium-rich vegetables are of special value. I put the patient to bed and have him fed such non-starchy vegetables as celery, parsley, zucchini, and string beans cooked in water and put through a blender. The patient is given nothing else until the urine becomes sugar-free. He remains in bed to conserve his energy and to give the liver and the pancreas every possible chance to do their work unmolested by the acids of exertion. It may take three or four days to get the patient sugar-free. Then he is placed on a careful diet and allowed to resume his regular routine, until he develops sugar in his urine again; then once more he is fasted on vegetable broth and finally given as ideal a diet for his particular case as possible.

Many thousands of words have been written about the value of raw versus cooked vegetables in the diet. The simplest rules to remember are that man and herbivorous animals must cook their vegetables in order to break down the cellulose (wood) box in which the vegetable cell is stored. Man uses heat; herbivorous animals use fermentation, for which they have separate stomachs. But to man, raw vegetables are also of great value, mainly for bulk and roughage as well as to keep the intestinal contents from becoming too dry. The human intestinal tract is so constructed that roughage is needed for rapid elimination of waste products and, equally important, for keeping the muscles strong. It must be remembered, of course, that when the intestinal lining is catarrhal or inflamed, rough-textured food often irritates or may even cause bleeding; hence, great discretion must be used with raw vegetables and fruits.

Discretion should be used as well in one's choice of vegetables. Today there are many machines on the market for the purpose of extracting the juice of vegetables, and they are becoming increasingly popular.

In addition to being mildly alkaline in reaction and containing some vitamins and trace elements, the most beneficial asset of raw vegetable juice is the type of water it contains. One might call this "natural water," most suited to the body's needs. This water is a much less irritating fluid than that which comes from the tap—chlorinated, perhaps fluoridated, and with, too often, a disagreeable taste and caustic action. The vegetable juices should be diluted with distilled water, if anything. Some vegetables contain pigments, such as the carotene of carrots, which may eventually turn the skin yellow. Green juices, as from parsley, spinach and other green leaves can be irritating to an inflamed intestinal lining, while the juice from red beets can turn the urine red. Great care must be used in their administration.

I am frequently asked about the value of a vegetarian diet. I do not advocate it as a way of life. While one cannot live comfortably in our environment *without* vegetables and fruits, one cannot live *entirely* on them and still *remain in a state of buoyant health.* I do, however, advocate a vegetable diet when the patient is "over-proteinized" after eating too much meat over a long period of time. When this happens, I place him on a vegetable diet until his tissues are free of too much stored animal protein. And then I suggest a diet with not too high a percentage of flesh, eggs and dairy products.

The controversy between meat eaters and vegetarians has raged for centuries and will, no doubt, continue. Many prominent persons have extolled vegetarianism on humanitarian grounds, notably the late George Bernard Shaw. Many, however, who call themselves "vegetarians" eat cheese, butter, eggs, and also drink milk; they are not "true" vegetarians but, rather, non-meat eaters. In that way, they remain on an excellent diet from the standpoint of nutrition.

In conclusion, there are several important points to remember about vegetables: It is best not to mix vegetables with fruit or other sweets at the same meal. Only one starchy vegetable should be eaten at a meal. Root vegetables, such as carrots, parsnips, turnips, beets, etc., do not digest well when cooked, as they have a tendency to create gas and acid fermentation. (These vegetables should not be confused with potatoes, which are tubers.) The combination of sugar, starch and proteins found in the legumes is most difficult for the sedentary person to digest, since they frequently create some intestinal disturbance. Vegetables should be steamed, preferably, or cooked in small amounts of water. Overcooking destroys enzymes and vitamins. Always use the cooking water, either in soups or as a drink. Remember that the volatile oils and other irritants found in onions, radishes, garlic, scallions, watercress, sharp-tasting salad greens, most spices and peelings with bitter flavors are poisons that nature puts into those plants to discourage the attacking insects. (In early days, spices were greatly sought after as preservatives or to cover the taste of tainted meat; today we have refrigeration.) Spices, then, are natural insecticides and therefore not edible, although often stimulating and appetite-whetting. But since these volatile oils may irritate the delicate kidney tubules, they should be eliminated from the diet. To those who use gourmet French cookbooks this will come as sad news; nevertheless, many of my colleagues and I believe it to be the truth.

17

Milk and Yeast as Food
and Medicine

The cows are our friends, they give food, they give strength, they likewise give a good complexion and happiness.

—GAUTAMA BUDDHA, 500 B.C.

MILK

In antiquity, priests of certain cultures made offerings of milk to their gods in a heaven thought of as a cow with full udder. Mankind's oldest food has a unique place in nutrition: it is the most nearly perfect of any *one* food and the best source of protein for adults as well as for infants and children. But because it tastes so good and goes down so easily, it is often taken in excessive amounts. Certainly, it should never be used merely to quench the thirst. Milk is a food, not a drink.

If the chemistry of the liver is normal, no harm is done when *raw* milk is taken as food, for the milk proteins are easily synthesized into our own body proteins. (You will note I said "raw"—not pasteurized.) But when the secretions of the liver are toxic and the bile is acid in reaction, trouble begins. It is also important to remember that milk is primarily the food for the growing calf, which doubles the weight of its bones every month for the first three months of its life, whereas the human infant needs six months to double its birth weight. To make this growth possible for the calf, cow's milk must and does contain a much higher calcium content than human milk. Dr. Henry C. Sherman of Columbia University, in his exhaustive studies of milk, found fifty-eight grains of calcium to the quart of cow's milk. He also demonstrated that the human growing child cannot utilize more than five grains a day. Again, for the calf's rapid growth, a much larger percentage of protein is needed; it is found in the casein of milk. This large amount of protein gives much energy to the calf. It can get along with a small amount of milk sugar but the human baby needs less protein and calcium and more sugar. These proportions are found in human milk. When we modify cow's milk for the infant we must keep this in mind. But why modify cow's milk? Isn't it time we rediscovered the mother's breast as the most perfect food source for her baby?

The average daily amount of cow's milk given to a baby up to six months should be one pint for each twenty-four hours. From six months until six years of age one and a half pints will prove adequate. But when other proteins such as eggs, cheese and meat are used, the amount of milk should be reduced accordingly. Another important fact to remember is that the liver is relieved of great strain if only *one* protein is taken at a meal. For instance, it is harmful to use milk or milk products at a meal where meat or fish or fowl is served. I cannot stress too highly that one protein at a time is the best rule.

If the liver secretions and bile are toxic and acid, the curd of milk, usually formed in the stomach, instead of being soft and flocculent, becomes as hard and tough as rubber and leads to much indigestion and constipation. The whey, being alkaline and full of calcium, neutralizes the acid bile, resulting in urate of lime, a muddy white substance which can clog the bile ducts, settle in the gall bladder and easily give rise to gallstones. This same substance gives the white coating to the tongue as well as the disagreeable odor from the mouth. (The strong odor of Limburger cheese comes from the putrefaction of the whey.)

It must be remembered that the tongue is the barometer of the liver. The type of coating, the edema, the inflammation of the various kinds of papillae and their eventual atrophy all indicate certain stages of liver damage. In liver disease we must be careful, therefore, how we use milk as a dietary protein, especially in older people. Dr. Leonard Williams of London made a sound observation when he remarked that a great many old people were floated into their coffins on milk.

Raw milk (or its constituent parts), when properly used, is one of the best nutrient proteins that can be offered as a rebuilder of body tissues. Hippocrates prescribed it for the treatment of tuberculosis. Dr. S. Wier Mitchell accomplished wonders in his practice and much of his therapy consisted of the milk diet combined with plenty of rest.

Many of the clinical states now classified as hypoadrenia (adrenal exhaustion) respond perfectly to the milk diet. And most milk-diet sanatoria stress the importance of much rest while taking milk at half-hour intervals. Four and a half to seven quarts are given daily. The milk is always fresh raw milk with most of the cream removed.

Dr. Charles S. Porter, who has given the milk-diet cure to thousands of patients, describes the subjective response of this diet:

Within two hours after commencing the diet, the action of the heart will be accelerated and within twelve to twenty-four hours there will be a gain of six beats to the minute. Within two or three days there will be an increase of about twelve beats to the minute; the pulse will be full and bounding; the skin flushed and moist; the capillary circulation quick and active ... There is an increase in the general warmth of the body ... The stimulation of a full milk diet is very similar to the effects of alcoholic stimulation on the circulation, but the aftereffects are entirely different ... The voluntary muscles of the body become firm and solid, almost like an athlete's limbs ... There is an increased power of the intestinal muscles, resulting in several copious bowel movements per day.

This is a perfect picture of what is called "adrenal response." But it must be remembered that a milk diet is not the "cure" for everyone. The response will depend upon the condition of the liver as indicated principally by the examination of the tongue and the urine.

The following case history describes my own clinical results with a patient suffering from advanced hypoadrenia. The patient, a sixty-four-year-old Missouri farmer, was too weak to sit up; he suffered greatly from cold and even with six hot water bottles his rectal temperature refused to go above ninety-three degrees. There was pallor of the skin, cyanosis of the fingernails, moderate dyspnea, advanced auricular fibrillation, pulse 72, blood pressure 100/90. There was also a great deal of intestinal gas, with such frequent eructations from the stomach that his rest was disturbed, and a moderate edema of the legs and feet, even while resting.

Treatment consisted of a diet of the curd of sweet raw milk mixed with finely chopped green lettuce; a teaspoonful every fifteen minutes the first two days and nights. Then the dose was gradually increased and given every half hour during fourteen hours of the day. His weight was 122 pounds. In two days he began to sleep and his heart was more regular, but he was still intensely cold. In five days he was warmer and the cyanosis was gone. In eleven days his edema had disappeared and his weight was 114, far too low for a man six-feet two-inches tall. In eighteen days he felt stronger, much warmer, and had no vertigo when erect. His nails were pink and the irregularity of the heart had almost entirely disappeared. Thirty-two days after the treatment was started, he returned to Missouri feeling well and strong. His weight went up to 121 pounds; in one month on the same diet he gained 27 pounds; a month later he weighed 153 pounds. Two years after treatment began, he was able to resume his farm work. The amount of curd had been gradually increased until he was taking the curd of seven quarts of milk daily. No other food was given except the lettuce.

When first seen, this patient was in a far advanced state of adrenal exhaustion. To whip what was left of his poor adrenals by giving salt solutions, stimulants or digitalis would have resulted in myocardial collapse. The protein colloids of the casein acted as a heart stimulant and simultaneously offered elements which the liver could utilize for general body repair. The adrenals gradually became recharged with phosphorus. And he made a complete recovery.

Raw milk is a good food and *sometimes* a good cure—that is, when used wisely. The Swiss, whose main protein is from milk and milk products, and the Masai, whose diet contains practically nothing else but milk and raw blood (they bleed as well as milk their cows) are among the healthiest and strongest people in the world.

Nature has taken great pains to insure the freshness of milk by the "nipple to mouth" delivery system. Indeed, the very chemical instability of milk makes for its easy digestibility. The Old Testament writers knew about this ease of digestion and exceptional nutritional qualities of milk when they said: "Such as have need of milk, and not of strong meat" (Hebrews V:12).

Unfortunately, man's various attempts to preserve milk have all resulted in altering or breaking down the complex molecule and reducing its value as a food. Far removed from the original formula are such deteriorations as buttermilk, dried milk powder, cheese and concentrated, pasteurized or homogenized milk. When the chief protein of the diet is composed of degenerated milk or milk products, the result is a maldeveloped mammal.

I have always prescribed raw milk and in my half century of practice have never seen a case of so-called "undulant" fever. Pasteurized milk putrefies in the intestines, whereas raw milk merely ferments. Indeed, pasteurized milk will putrefy in the bottle, when placed in a warm room, and will be a smelly mess in four or five days; raw milk will only ferment and be edible as clabber.

It has always been known that the fresher the raw milk, the more valuable its quality as food. Mr. Richard Dawson, a California dairyman, reported an experiment illustrating this fact. When cows gave birth to twin calves in his dairy, one calf was allowed to suckle the mother and the other was "bucket-fed." The bucket milk was raw but had been chilled and was from twelve to twenty-four hours old. As the calves developed, the difference in growth was plainly apparent. As much as four inches difference in height was noted, and the bucket-fed calf was less vigorous and lacked the glossy coat of the former. That pasteurization of milk can result in a deterioration fatal to animals was shown by Dr. Pottenger in his cat experiments. John Thomson of Edinburgh reports another test with twin calves, one suckled and the other fed on pasteurized milk. The first was healthy but the second died within sixty days. This experiment was repeated many times.

The statement of Hippocrates, "Thy food shall be thy remedy," is as applicable today as it was centuries ago. In view of the milk processors and innovators of new forms of preserving milk by powdering or concentrating it, another aphorism of Hippocrates is equally timely: "For they praise what is outlandish before they know whether it is good, rather than the customary which they already know to be good; the bizarre, rather than the obvious."

YEAST

Yeasts, among the first forms of vegetable life on our planet, probably came into human use by a happy accident. Yeast cells very likely came in contact with the wild-grain paste a primitive housewife was preparing one hot day, expanded when heated on hot stones and produced lightened or leavened bread. Another happy discovery soon was made: a bit of this dough would carry the magic leavening property to a new batch of grain paste. In time, a yeast pot became a family's treasured possession and a bride carried her own yeast pot to her new home.

But we are concerned with yeast as a food. Because of its mild alkalinity, yeast is soothing to inflamed surfaces and absorbs and neutralizes acids. It is one of the most valuable antidotes against acid or toxic bile. As a source of the B vitamins it is unexcelled. R. H. A. Plummer of London has shown its ability to enhance normal carbohydrate digestion and to prevent the accumulation of incompletely oxidized fatty acids, such as pyruvic, lactic and acetic acids, all of which are so detrimental to body tissues. Acid or toxic bile often irritates the small intestine enough to cause spasms which block the normal peristaltic waves. This is one of the most common causes of constipation. Yeast, being alkaline, neutralizes the irritation in the bowels and is capable of restoring normal bowel movements, but it cannot be classified as a laxative.

Yeast has a beneficial effect on the skin, and has long been used as a remedy for pimples and acne. Vitamins in yeast help the deranged liver to oxidize fats in the diet properly. It is the incompletely oxidized fats in the diet that clog the oil and sebaceous glands and thus cause acne. Although eating yeast will remedy acne and pimples, it may be necessary also to eliminate fats from the diet, especially butter, other shortenings, cream and fatty cheeses. I understand that yeast mixed with a little rosewater makes an excellent and inexpensive facial mask for the ladies.

In addition to its use for skin disorders, yeast is useful for ulcer sufferers. It is soft in the intestines, alkaline, non-corrosive and non-irritating. For patients with bleeding gastric ulcers, when even squash or string bean vegetable broth of the best kind would be too caustic to put over an ulcer, yeast, diluted in a little milk or water, is helpful. I have given as many as twenty-two cakes a day to such patients and in a few days the ulcer has healed. Generally, I suggest two or three cakes a day to many of my patients—one early in the morning because it is a great buffer against acid bile. When one wakes up with a bilious hangover, a yeast cake in a little hot water will sweeten the digestive system and afford three times as much benefit from breakfast. The taste is agreeable, somewhat like cheese, and the aftertaste is most refreshing.

Occasionally, people complain of intestinal gas after taking yeast. This is mainly due to bowel stasis and stagnation. The continued use of yeast will finally result in the complete disappearance of gas. But persons who are nauseated by yeast or who find its taste disagreeable should not try to take it; they should seek alkaline antidotes from other members of the vegetable kingdom.

There are two varieties of yeast on the market. Fresh, compressed, soft baker's yeast, which can be obtained in one-pound blocks from most bakeries, keeps well in the refrigerator. There are also small cakes, wrapped in foil; this size, though, even when refrigerated, is highly perishable. After a few days, it becomes hard, moldy or spotted with fungus, bitter to the taste and disagreeable to the stomach. These tiny cakes are often too old to use when purchased. Recently, this type of yeast has been made available dried in fine granular form and packaged in small cellophane bags. Like the block or cake yeast, it is "alive," meaning that it is useful for the leavening of dough. It also has advantages for direct consumption; it keeps well at room temperature and can be carried on trips into countries where it is unobtainable.

The second variety is brewer's yeast. This preparation has lately been popularized by the writer of a bestselling book on living the long life. This yeast is reduced to a powder by being sprayed through drying chambers kept at a temperature of 250 degrees Fahrenheit—much the same as milk has been reduced to an indigestible powder—which kills and sterilizes it. It keeps well, but is classed as a "dead" yeast because it will not leaven dough. The heating not only reduces the vitamin content but also changes its organic salts into inorganic salts, which are less easily used by the body. The heating also renders it acid, therefore stimulating, and gives it a "chicken soup" flavor. Unlike the fresh yeast, it is compatible with any kind of food and causes less flatulence. Although not as potent a product as live yeast, it has some value and is better than no yeast at all.

Yeast is a vegetable, composed of minute cells about the size of red corpuscles, loosely held together like a bunch of grapes. They differ from other plant cells because they are not surrounded by a cellulose box which must be destroyed before the cell can be useful as food. Cooking breaks down this cellulose box; man cooks his vegetables in a pot; herbivorous animals cook their food in their first stomachs, which are fermentation vats. But the end results are the same. The naked yeast cells are easily acted upon by the digestive juices and for that reason are readily absorbed. Cooking partially destroys the vitamins of yeast cells. In their raw state, they are the richest source of the B vitamins and are also rich in alkaline elements, especially sodium and potassium. As noted earlier, they have a most valuable buffer reaction against stomach, liver and intestinal acids.

Even before the vitamins were discovered it was believed that yeast had therapeutic value, especially as a remedy for indigestion, heartburn and constipation. But yeast did not really become popular until Prohibition. Strangely enough, the company that put the product on the market, with full-page advertisements, really performed a disservice for users of this valuable product. They were urged to take yeast with fruit juices, especially orange or tomato juice, or to spread it on bread or crackers. The result was an increased amount of fermentation in stomach and bowels. Instead of drinking beer, yeast-eaters, mixing the yeast with juice, manufactured beer in their stomachs and bowels—with the attendant pleasure of alcoholic fermentation. But fusel oils, toxic alcohols and acids, harmful to the liver and kidneys, were also by-products.

Later, it was found that these toxic by-products had a detrimental effect on the vitamins of the yeast. Today, one school of dietetics condemns fresh, live yeast for that very reason and recommends brewer's yeast as a substitute. Instead of concluding that "here is a bad food combination," these so-called authorities decided that fresh yeast itself is harmful and should therefore be condemned. It is to be regretted that having come so close to a logical explanation of improper food chemistry, the facts could be so twisted out of reason.

Fresh yeast, although far superior to brewer's yeast, should not be ingested except when the stomach is empty. It should be eaten by itself, allowed to dissolve slowly in the mouth, or mixed with warm water or milk—never with anything else. The best times to take fresh yeast are early in the morning or one hour before the evening meal or at bedtime. It may be repeated during the night. I have used it for nearly half a century in my practice and have never seen any harmful effects when used in this manner. Occasionally, in special cases, it may be taken after meals free from sugars or starches for the relief of stomach pain or heartburn.

Finally, it must be remembered that the liver is the largest and most important organ in the body and that one of its chief functions is to strain toxins and impurities from the blood stream. As long as the liver is normal, the blood stream remains pure; disease, therefore, is impossible. The result of improper diet is to break down the liver, reducing its alkalinity by robbing it of its organic sodium. One of the first symptoms of liver impairment is fatigue, a common complaint of Americans. For the neutralization of liver toxicity, sodium-rich vegetables are needed. Yeast, at a few pennies a cake, may be called the poor man's sodium-rich vegetable. Let me say again that it is one of the richest sources of natural organic vitamins and a powerful antidote against toxic bile. When bad food habits have been eliminated, yeast should always have a prominent place in the recuperative diet. Used therapeutically, it is one of the most valuable of foods.

18

Salt and Stimulation vs. the Good Diet

> Now learn what and how great benefits a temperate
> diet will bring along with it. In the first place, you will
> enjoy good health.
>
> —HORACE, 65–8 B.C.

To be of real service to the patient, the physician must diagnose the patient's disease before its ravages have laid waste his vital organs. Diseases must be diagnosed in their incipiency, long before there are organic signs and symptoms; often before there are marked functional disturbances. How can this be done? The only chance to do this is through a better understanding of the body chemistry, which includes the chemistry and functions of the endocrine glands. Because it is food which makes the blood and it is the blood which in turn feeds the cells, it is necessary also to know something of the chemistry of food and digestion if we are to remain in good health. What constitutes nutrition, and what is the difference between nutrition and stimulation? How often is a condition of so-called health really a mask of stimulation beneath which the vital organs are being destroyed?

Food, to sustain life and health and to permit growth, must be *organic* in form. *Inorganic* substances, even though used in small quantities, stimulate but at the same time may also poison insidiously. In larger doses or with prolonged use these same inorganic substances (usually used for seasonings and to enhance the normal flavor of foods) may cause deterioration of vital organs. The inorganic substance most commonly used is, of course, sodium chloride—common table salt.

Long ago it was observed that in certain states of body deterioration, salt seemed to aggravate the condition. Now we know that it interferes with the elimination of certain waste products of metabolism. In earlier days, it was noted that the patient with kidney disease became edematous (filled with fluid), a direct result of having too much salt in the blood. Controlled experiments revealed that sodium chloride interfered with the elimination of uric acid products, thus aggravating the symptoms of such diseases as rheumatism and eczema. And later it was proved, again by controlled experiments on dogs and chickens—who eliminate a good deal of nitrogen as uric acid—that the result of feeding salt, even in very small quantities, was death. Autopsy revealed the liver and kidneys of these animals and birds to be studded with uric acid concretions precipitated by the salt.

Yet, what is the most common argument advanced *for* salt eating? Why, of course, that animals have long been known to travel great distances, if necessary, to obtain salt from salt licks. But how do we know that these animals are not mineral-starved and lick salt as a poor substitute for browsing on leaves and twigs? Even when we give the horse plenty of salt, he still chews the bark off trees, gnaws his manger board and rasps the telephone poles. Does the fact that animals *like* salt mean that they need it? Does an obese woman need a hot fudge sundae because she likes it? Introduce a horse to sugar, then give him his choice between a sugar mash and a salt mash. He will gorge himself on the sugar mash and ignore the salt mixture. Does that mean that horses need sugar? At best, the argument is most flimsy and does not merit consideration except for the fact that salt is a stimulant. It makes us feel good by elevating the blood pressure a little and stimulating the adrenal glands. This stimulation brings a happier mental state and a feeling of warmth, alertness and seeming good health. Over and over we read that salt is necessary for life. But is it? Dr. Benjamin Rush found the American Indians he studied as healthy as Stefansson found the Eskimos or as Bartholomew found the peoples of interior China—yet none of them ever ate salt.

Salt, man's earliest condiment, was considered sacred by the Romans and there is no country which does not have its hoard of salt superstitions and maxims. Throughout history, salt has been considered a potent medicine and used therapeutically. In small doses, it acts as a stimulant; in large doses it is an embalming fluid. The ancient Egyptians used oils, spices and *salt* in their mummy wrappings; today we mummify the *living* with salad dressings made of oils, spices and *salt*. A walk along any street discloses its share of these mummies; the dry skin, shrunken bodies and white hair, outward symbols of hardened livers and sclerotic kidneys. As I observe them, I often wonder why it is necessary to embalm such salt-filled bodies after they are dead.

"The amount of sodium chloride taken in the form of common salt is far in excess of human requirements for sodium and chlorine," declared nutritionist Mary Swartz Rose, Ph.D., in *Foundations of Nutrition*. "Furthermore, these elements are so widely distributed in food materials that there is little likelihood of shortage of either unless some specially restricted diet is employed over a long period of time or one is working under conditions of excessive heat. The main question is whether or not sodium chloride will be used to excess." Personally, I disagree with the late Dr. Rose on the need for more salt for workers in hot climates, as I will explain in this chapter.

Why is salt so harmful? When taken in small doses it is immediately eliminated from the body through the sweat and urine. In larger doses, it is retained in the body tissues and blood stream, resulting in a state of hyperchloremia, which means that a super-normal amount is circulating in the blood stream. Salt, in this amount, distinctly stimulates the individual. And if, in this state of stimulation, a rapid sweating occurs, the amount of salt in the blood would be suddenly lowered, resulting in a state of hypochloremia. This sudden drop of the salt content of the blood depresses the user. Not only has the stimulant been removed but the isotonic equilibrium of the blood stream and body cells has suddenly been upset, resulting in a shock to the body tissues, especially to the more sensitive nerve and brain tissues. If, in this state of hypochloremia, salt is ingested, the individual regains an equilibrium, is stimulated and feels normal again. In short, a state of chemical disequilibrium has been restored; or a so-called "cure" for the weakness has been effected.

This explains the apparent value of salt tablets recommended by many medical men, and especially by salt-tablet manufacturers, for use in hot weather.

It is possible for a person to eliminate salt quite rapidly through channels such as the skin and kidneys. As long as the body is strong, the resistance good and the glands of internal secretion adequate, not much salt is retained. But when the channels of elimination are inadequate, salt retention results, with its attendant harmful consequences. This happens in three stages generally: in the first, the liver or kidneys or skin, or all three, may show functional derangement, followed (second stage) by organic destruction. Albumen, casts, red blood cells and pus in the urine—all signs of extensive kidney destruction—may usher in the third stage of salt poisoning. The second stage may consist of the transient occurrence of albumen in the urine after moderate exercise or an unusually heavy meal. In the first stage, the excess of NaCl in the urine (which causes no signs or symptoms) begins even while a person feels well and considers himself healthy. But by the time the third stage is reached, the kidneys are so impaired that salt elimination is greatly interfered with. It may be too late then to accomplish very much for the patient by restricting salt in the diet. Somewhere along the line there was a point at which salt began to be dangerous. The railroads have found that the best way to eliminate dangerous crossings is to eliminate crossings; so the public crosses the tracks on overhead bridges or underground, through subways, and stays off the tracks.

The eating of inorganic salt is a bad habit. Why not, then, let the plants synthesize NaCl into an organic form, in their leaves and fruits and roots and stems, and eat it that way? A simple solution, isn't it? *The urine and sweat never show an excess of salt when it is consumed in this form.*

There are other stimulants, such as coffee, tobacco, alcohol and morphine, which can become concentrated in the blood and body tissues. These, too, when suddenly discontinued, result in violent upsets to the nervous equilibrium. When the average healthy young person drinks coffee regularly, he eliminates the coffee acids through the urine soon after he drinks it. And it has no deleterious effects. The beverage affords him a certain amount of stimulation and a feeling of all's-well-with-the-world. But as the kidneys gradually deteriorate with advancing age, there comes a time when coffee acids are not eliminated shortly after the coffee is drunk. Drop by drop then, they pile up in the system. And the healthy man does not feel so healthy and he decides to discontinue coffee. Instead of feeling better instantly, he finds himself wracked with a constant and violent headache. He is surprised when told that he is suffering withdrawal symptoms, milder to be sure, but still symptoms like those a narcotics addict suffers.

The headache following coffee withdrawal persists for the length of time it takes the coffee poisons to be eliminated. They leave the system in a high concentration that may take from one day up to two weeks. If, then, he cuts his coffee-drinking to a safe margin, he will eliminate the harmful coffee acids through urination. Sooner or later, however, he will find such elimination impossible and the toxic acids build up in his body. For a time coffee continues to stimulate, then he begins to find that he needs an extra cup several times a day as a pick-up. That is why the "coffee break" habit is so pernicious—it offers extra coffee to people who should not be drinking it in such large amounts.

After the body is made toxic by a high concentration of coffee poisons over a long period of time, coffee ceases to stimulate, no matter how much is drunk, and a period of depression follows. It is a dangerous period, I believe, for the body is saturated with poisons and very fatigued, precisely the time when some sort of health catastrophe may occur—arthritis, neuritis, cancer.

Long before such health breakdowns occur, it is noted that coffee, when abruptly discontinued, results in many people in headaches which can be "cured" by drinking more coffee. The alcoholic, when his stimulant is suddenly withdrawn, may develop delirium tremens, the cure for which is more alcohol. The cigarette addict, too, rushes to the foyer during the intermission of a theatrical performance in a nervous haste to light up again. The narcotics addict, when suddenly deprived of his support, collapses and is "restored" by doses of his drug. All of which simply proves that the chemical equilibrium of the body cannot be changed suddenly without upsetting the individual. But these are not proofs that coffee *cures* headaches; that tobacco *cures* nervousness; that alcohol *cures* delirium tremens or that morphine *cures* depression.

But, to return to our discussion of salt stimulation. The foreman who is undertaking a job during extremely hot weather or in an oppressive atmosphere requires efficiency on the part of his workmen. If by feeding them large amounts of salt in the form of salt tablets he can maintain this efficiency so that the job gets done in the specified time, then he is all for feeding them salt. Whether any chemical harm is being done to the internal organs of his workers does not concern him. Bright's disease, arteriosclerosis, anemia, mucous membrane inflammations are all too remote to worry him. He's no scientist, so he sees no connection between those diseases and a state of chronic salt poisoning, although the medical profession currently believes that Bright's disease, arteriosclerosis, high blood pressure, asthma and hay fever are all relieved by a salt-free diet.

The activity of goldfish in an aquarium is increased by adding salt to the water. Observing them in vigorous motion, it is easy to believe they are in excellent health although the salt has merely stimulated them. Actually it is easy to confuse a state of stimulation with a state of health. Even doctors can be confused and sometimes prescribe stimulants indiscriminately. But the inevitable breakdown proves the inconsistency of stimulative therapy.

The late British heart specialist, Sir James Mackenzie, observed that, "The first appearance of disease in the human body is invariably insidious with little disturbance of the economy and no visible signs of its presence. By and by the patient becomes conscious that all is not well with him; there is a loss of that feeling of well-being which accompanies the healthy state. Disagreeable sensations arise, at first vague but later becoming more definite and these may become so urgent that he seeks advice. Still no evident sign of disease may be perceived on the most careful examination. By and by the disease, being situated in some organ or tissue, changes the constitution of that part so that its presence is now recognized by a physical sign, when the clinical methods usually employed reveal its character."

Only by careful chemical examination of secretions, such as mucus, tears, gastric juice, urine, joint fluids, spinal fluid and blood, can we arrive at early diagnoses of salt poisoning. Our figures for the normal blood chlorides are all too high, it seems to me, since most of the so-called normal cases were early cases of salt retention. Again, to quote Mackenzie: "There are evidences which would surely indicate the nature of the disease in its earliest stages, were we capable of detecting them."

Here, I should like to offer my own ideas, researched over the years, on stimulation versus good health: Addiction to alcohol, tobacco, coffee and tea, stimulating drugs, salt, pepper, spices of all kinds and synthetic vitamins are stimulation habits which, sooner or later, lower energy and destroy health. The individual who shakes salt vigorously over his dinner without even tasting it, the one who fortifies himself nightly with several cocktails before eating an enormous steak for dinner and follows that up with cup after cup of coffee, does so because he momentarily feels better after-wards. If you take away his stimulating food or salt or drugs he is likely to feel weak, headachy, fatigued and depressed. His work may suffer. Assuming that this state will be habitual with him, he is, understandably, fearful and decides that dietary reform is for the birds.

He does not realize that his stimulating habits, whether of food or drugs, make him feel better *because he is whipping his endocrine glands*, most usually the adrenal glands, to produce an effect of exhilaration that merely masks his underlying fatigue. Just how long can he continue to mistreat his body?

Certainly, the public should be educated in this matter of stimulation habits about which so little is heard. But, unhappily, there are many, many people in this country who could not be helped even if they were reachable. In the South, for instance, there are thousands of people so overworked, so curtailed in life and born with such a weak body structure, glandularly and physically, that if they didn't continue to stimulate themselves by their atrocious vitamin-deficient diet of pork and salt and grease and white sugar and hot bread and corn likker and coffee, they couldn't work enough to keep up even their wretched standard of living. Not only are coffee, salt, sugar and corn whiskey stimulating and warming to the body, but so are pork, bacon grease, hot bread and pie—and all of them are equally successful in masking chronic fatigue temporarily. So they continue with their stimulation habits until, still young, they deteriorate to the point where work is impossible. Fortunately, many children today are being better fed in the South: whole-wheat bread, milk and wider use of well-cooked vegetables and fresh fruits are taking the place of turnip and mustard greens boiled all day with fat salt pork. Thus, nutritional advice in public schools is paving the way, slowly to be sure, to better health.

When we study the skulls of men of earlier times, we find the ivory of their teeth in excellent condition even though the skulls have deteriorated. At that period, the diet consisted of 80 percent vegetables which accounts for the beautiful and perfectly erupted teeth. Today we are lucky if the diet contains 5 percent of vegetables and, of course, the rest of the health of the body is in the same ratio.

Is, then, the witty Dr. Herbert Ratner exaggerating when he says: Modern man ends up a vitamin-taking, antacid-consuming, barbiturate-sedated, aspirin-alleviated, Benzedrine-stimulated, psychosomatically diseased, surgically despoiled animal; nature's highest product turns out to be a fatigued, peptic-ulcerated, tense, headachy, overstimulated, neurotic, tonsil-less creature.

Equally thought-provoking is Dr. Ratner's candid comment: "I showed a former dean of our medical school a talk I had prepared. When he came to [the above line] he said, 'Gee, Herb, I wish you'd not use that line. It will antagonize the drug-houses, and we are trying to build up research funds.'"

Over and over, I am asked: "What, then, is the *right* diet?" when I have pointed out the relation of poor food habits to disease. And although most members of the medical profession are opposed to the idea that food can possibly have anything to do with instigating disease states, many physicians, as I have pointed out previously, ask me to recommend a good diet for cancer or arthritis and other chronic diseases when they see the success I have achieved with seriously ill patients. It is impossible to answer these questions specifically without knowing the glandular balance, the chemistry, the heredity, the habits and the impaired functions of the organs regulating the person's digestion. Much as I wish I could be of service, I find I cannot, in good conscience, accommodate these medical men.

It is known, for instance, that man needs proteins, fats, starches, sugars, roughage, vitamins, organic salts and water. Some of these foods are much more easily digested than others. So let me simplify this list in an attempt to select the very best and most easily digestible and least harmful of foods. Let me warn, though, that the list is narrow and allows little chance for variety or for daily dining in fashionable French restaurants. But the healthful state following the use of these foods more than compensates for their monotony.

Among the most easily digestible proteins are *rare beef and lamb, raw or lightly cooked egg yolks and fresh raw unpasteurized milk.* The reason the meat should be rare, or as near raw as the person can eat it, is explained elsewhere in this book as is also the use of egg yolk and milk. Vegetable proteins, such as nuts, avocadoes and legumes, are valuable but classed as second-rate proteins. As for fats, the most ideal is butterfat. Meat and vegetable fats have their uses but are second-rate. The boiled (preferably steamed) white potato heads the list of useful starches. Cereal starches come next, followed by raw cane sugar and the natural sugars of fruits. Roughage is exceedingly important because of the anatomy of man's intestines; the least irritating varieties are leaves, stalks, stems, and the solid parts of fruits and vegetables.

An important point to remember is that when the food elements mentioned above are included in the diet, there is no need for extra vitamins and organic salts. For instance, Stefansson clearly demonstrated that fresh raw or rare-cooked meat contained all of the vitamins and organic salts needed to insure perfect health.

Now, let us take a look at the man who is going to eat these foodstuffs. Even though he uses the best forms of sugars and starches, their digestion may be impaired by an imperfect chemistry of his *own* saliva, pancreas and small intestine. Proteins may encourage tumors or cancers; fats may cause boils or carbuncles; sugars supply acidity and flatulence; roughage may result in diarrhea and hemorrhage; vitamins and organic salts may cause a harmful stimulation. Any of these ailments may afflict people who are suffering from various forms of toxemia, the vicarious elimination of which greatly interferes with the proper chemistry of the digestive juices and the bile. Here, too, is a clear demonstration of that old cliché: One man's meat is another man's poison. Here we see, also, the impossibility of writing a book filled with dietary recipes.

Sometimes it is important to refrain from eating and thus give the exhausted digestive system a short rest, as I have demonstrated in cases from my files. The digestion becomes so impaired, so limited, that only one or two foods can be tolerated. Let me cite an example. A man came to me suffering from shortness of breath and swelling of the legs. He was a political boss, powerful, well-loved by his constituents. Examination disclosed an extreme debilitation of the heart, and also showed that he was unable to handle sugars, starches, or fats. It was also found that the only time during the twenty-four-hour span when he was able to digest or assimilate anything was during the hours from 11 A.M. to 2 P.M.

Essentially his treatment was simple. He was taken off all drugs and given one meal at noon daily, consisting of rare ground beef mixed with chopped lettuce and celery and then lightly broiled.

Depending on his hunger, he would eat from half to a pound of meat. In three weeks his dropsy, weakness and shortness of breath disappeared. He resumed his active political life. I told him many times how allergic he was to sugars and starches and I warned him repeatedly that the slightest ingestion of such food might prove fatal. His good health continued for over two years. Then, during a birthday celebration by his constituents, a huge, festive birthday cake was brought in. He declined to sample it but his friends literally forced him to join them. He ate a large slice. Within twenty-four hours, he was dead. Of course, I need not add that this is an extreme example of food allergy.

When the digestive juices become toxic or impaired, the chemistry of digestion is always interfered with. And this is what Hippocrates meant when he spoke of "vicious humors." The bile and pancreatic juice pour into the small intestine a few inches below the stomach and mix with ingested food. Both of these may be "vicious humors." They may especially interfere with certain combinations of even the best of foods.

Books on various diets fill many shelves in the libraries. "As old as the story of Adam and the apple is man's belief in the specificity of certain foods," comments the *Journal of the American Dietetic Association*. "There will always be those who, with specious reasoning, would claim to have divined the elixir of youth in some one food or very limited group of foods. The realm of nutrition and dietetics, unfortunately, has always been and probably always will be a happy hunting ground for those who would pervert scientific findings to their own advantage." Personal observations have led many food faddists to conclude that certain food combinations are dangerous. For example, it is commonly said that starch and protein is a bad combination. What these faddists miss seeing is that starch and protein and *toxic bile* form a bad combination. As most diet books are based on personal idiosyncrasies and prejudices, the usual result is an amazing collection of good and bad combinations. Nature, in her wisdom, has never created a food which is entirely protein, starch or sugar. Even meat contains relatively large amounts of starch (as glycogen and muscle sugar).

Therefore, the best I can do in prescribing diets is to give a fair amount of digestible food to the patient while trying to neutralize his toxemia with vegetable or fruit antidotes. Too many food fads and dietary restrictions among great leaders or powerful men have had their effect upon the masses. For example, a French king suffered asthma attacks during the night. So his physicians concluded that "night air" was bad for him. Immediately his subjects decided that "night air" was bad for them.

Perhaps Sir William Osler was thinking of food fads when he remarked: "We are all dietetic sinners; only a small percent of what we eat nourishes us, the balance goes to waste and loss of energy." Equally observant is this comment, with its hint of sly humor: "Most of what we eat is superfluous. Hence, we only live off a quarter of all we swallow: Doctors live off the other three quarters." Sounds very modern, doesn't it? Well, it was inscribed on an ancient Egyptian papyrus! From antiquity to today, man has ever searched hungrily for the "good diet."

Let me repeat: there are about as many amino acids—the building blocks of body protein—as there are letters in the alphabet. The thousands of words in the largest dictionary are composed of the twenty-six letters; the thousands of different protein combinations in body cells come from the small number of amino acids. This is why every human being has a different scent to the delicate nose of a dog and why the mother seal knows her own baby when it is surrounded by hundreds of baby seals. The ability to digest is often colored by the chemistry of the body protein itself.

Although I have tried to stress in this book the importance of knowing what to eat and what not to eat, the reader should remember that it is often more important to know *when not to eat at all.* A short fast on diluted fruit or vegetable juices gives an ill person a welcome opportunity to eliminate his toxic wastes. If, then, the blood chemistry is altered by the proper selection of food, the person will be restored to health.

Finally, much investigation remains to be done in the broad relation between diet and the occurrence of disease. Much investigation also remains to be done concerning human nutritional needs. At present we do not fully understand those needs. But we do know that the preferred source of nutrition is food, as fresh and natural as can be obtained, not dead products standing on drug-store shelves.

Index

Abscesses, 107
Acetic acid, 146
Acne, 102, 106, 214
Acromegaly, *see* Gigantism
Addison's disease, 71, 83
Adrenal glands, xv, 8, 43, 44, 45, 47,
  70, 74, 89, 90, 122–23, 130, 133,
  135, 151, 165, 168, 171, 184, 197,
  198, 212, 224
Adrenal-type body, 83–86, 87, 92,
  95, 141, 151
Alcohol, 46, 222, 223, 224, 225
Alimentary canal, 55, 61
Allergy, 7, 228
Ameboid movement, 58
American Dietetic Association, 18
Amino acids, 56, 57, 58, 59, 78–79,
  177, 179, 180, 181, 229
Anemia, 223
Aneurism, 115
Antibiotic Age, xiii
Antibiotics, 7, 9, 39, 109, 158, 159,
  168
Antigens, 7
Appendicitis, 47, 157–63
Appendectomy, 157–58
Arteriosclerosis, 39, 115, 223
Arthritis, 19–20, 47, 128, 192, 205
Ascites, 67
Asheville, North Carolina, 195
Aspirin, 107, 172
Assimilation, 179
Asthma, 163–65, 223, 229
Atherosclerosis, 115
Atlas of Men (Sheldon), 82
Atoms, 178
Aureomycin, 159

Bacteria, 31, 43, 159

Bagehot, Walter, 50
Barker, Lewellyn, 70
Beaumont, William, 57
Bicknell, Franklin, 159
Bile, 62, 65–66, 111, 112, 145, 192,
  208, 213, 214, 227, 228
Bile burn spasms, 66
Billings, John Shaw, 38
Biochemistry, 49
Bladder, 130
Blindness, 45, 46
Blood pressure, 135–37, 140–41, 223;
  see also Hypertension
Blood vessels, 60
Body, the human, 14–28, 30–31, 42,
  54–55, 78, 187, 196; adrenal type,
  83–86, 87, 92, 95, 141, 151; pitui-
  tary type, 88–89, 95–96; thyroid
  type, 86–88, 94–95, 155
Body-typing, 81–96
Boerhaave, Hermann, 8, 12, 40, 49
Boils, 43, 102, 107, 147, 227
Bonds, 117
Boyle, Robert, 31
Bright's disease, 223
Bronchitis, 47; of the lungs, 74
Buddha, *quoted*, 208
Buerger's disease, 118–19
Bursitis, 47
Butterfat, 114

Calcium, 204, 209
Calories, 149, 186, 201
Cancer, 20–21, 39, 101, 172, 174,
  189, 199, 205, 227
Carbohydrates, 55, 57, 60, 186, 196
Carbuncles, 43, 102, 147, 227
Carrel, Alexis, 153
Casein, 209

Catarrhs, 43
Cells, body, 31, 33, 40, 43, 57, 178, 180-81
Cellulose, 205, 215
Cervantes, Miguel de, 199
Cervicitis, 47
Charles II, of England, 33
Chicken pox, 107
Childhood diseases, 99-112
Chlorophyll vegetables, 203
Cholesterol, xv, 49-50, 113-28
Cirrhosis of the liver, 66, 192
Clark, Marguerite, quoted, 3
Clendening, Logan, 51
Cod liver oil theory, 6
Coffee, 222-23, 224, 225
Cold, the common, 8-9, 165-69, 198,
Colloids, 178, 191, 196
Conrad, Joseph, 60
Constipation, 56, 197
Coronary thrombosis, 115, 118
Cortex, 70-71
Corticoids, 6
Cortisone, 133
"Cradle cap," 106
Croups, 198
Cushing's disease, 91
Cyanide poisoning, 47

Dairy products, 196
Dark Age of Medicine, xiii
Davis, Adele, 155
Dawson, Richard, 212
Degenerative diseases, 31, 38, 182
Dehydration, 134-35
De La Mare, Walter, 155-56
Delirium tremens, 223
Dermatitis, 128
Dewey, James Hooker, 155
Diabetes, 39, 128, 169-70, 205
Diarrhea, 56, 60, 193, 227
Diet, What It Is and What It Isn't (Gibson), 194
Dietetics, 228
Diets, 38, 77-78, 81, 94, 99, 115-16, 125-26, 144, 146, 147, 148-52, 170, 178, 183, 186, 188, 206, 210-11, 226-30
Digestion, 6, 26, 54-61, 179, 180, 193, 212, 227

Diptheria, 39, 101, 107
Diseases, 29-35, 46-47, 157-74, 189, 205, 218, 223-24; causes of, 31-35, 42, 51, 52, 102, 157; childhood, 99-112; classes of, 31; degenerative, 31, 38, 182; germ theory of, xiv, 38-39, 40-41, 102; infectious, 31, 39; see also under name and type of disease
Doctors, Patients and Health Insurance (Somers), 33
Donaldson, Blake F., 147, 148
Don Quixote (Cervantes), 199
Dropsy, 138, 140-41
Drug addiction, 4
Drug reaction, adverse, 4-5, 9, 158-59
Drugs, xiii-xiv, 4-13, 18, 25, 38, 39, 51, 59, 93, 109, 133, 158, 200, 224
Dwarfism, 88

Ectomorphs, 82
Eczema, 46
Edema, 138, 140-41
Eisenhower, Dwight D., 124
Electrocardiograph, 126-28
Elimination of toxins, 4-5, 174; emergency vicarious, 42-49
Emerson, Ralph Waldo, 112
Encephalitis, 47
Endocrine glands, xiv, 8, 43-44, 45, 69-76, 82, 83, 101, 171, 174, 218, 224; see also Adrenal glands; Pituitary gland; Thyroid gland
Endocrine obesity type, 149, 150-53
Endocrinology, 82-83, 90, 94
Endomorphs, 82
Enteritis, 47
Enzymes, 55, 207
Epidemics, 33
Epilepsy, 45, 89, 205
Eskimos, 115-16, 183, 189-90, 220

Fasting, total, 104, 144-46, 229
Fats, 55, 57, 60, 100, 112, 115-19, 141, 186, 187, 196, 203, 226, 227
Fatty acids, 56, 102, 147, 213
Feeding the infant, 109-12, 197-98, 209
Fermentation, 205, 207, 215

Fever, 42, 107–09
Fischer, Martin H., 27, 139
Fish, 189, 190
Fletcher, Horace, 147
Food, as best medicine, 36–37; good
    diet, the, 226–30; inorganic sub-
    stances as, 218–19; milk, 208–13;
    natural, 182–83; overindulgence of,
    obesity type, 149–50; processes,
    concentrated and synthesized, 66;
    proteins as body builders, 177–85;
    proteins as body killers, 186–99;
    quality of, 57; quantity of, 56–57;
    stimulants, 218–26; stimulating ef-
    fects of, 44; vegetables, 200–07;
    yeast, 213–17; see also Diets
Fruits, 201, 206, 227, 229

Galen, 14, 72
Gastritis, 47, 192
Genesis and Control of Disease, The
    (Weger), 49
Germs, xiv, 31, 38, 39, 40, 53, 102,
    147, 168
Germ theory, xiv, 38–39, 40–41, 102
Gibson, Axel Emil, 194
Gigantism (acromegaly), 45, 46, 83,
    88
Glands, 43; of external secretion, 69;
    of internal secretion, 69; see also
    under name of gland
Glandular imbalance, 174
Glucose, 56, 60
Goiter, 74
Goldblatt, Harry, 136–37
Goode, Ruth, 62
Gouernayle of Helthe, 202

Habits of eating, 17–18
Harvey, William, quoted, 36
Hay fever, 171–72, 223
Heart, 6, 26, 119–22, 124
Heart Attack, (Prinzmetal), 125
Heart disease, 26, 39, 113–28, 189
Hemorrhage, 66, 123, 124, 227
Hepatitis, 39, 128, 205
Herber, Louis, 51–52
Hippocrates, 3, 11–12, 14, 19, 32,
    39, 41, 49, 57, 82, 144, 169, 183,
    204, 213, 228
Hippocratic Oath, 3

Hoffman, Frederick, 20–21
Hollywood Eighteen Day Diet, 149
Holmes, Oliver Wendell, 11, 197
Holt, L. Emmett, Jr., 187–88
Hooton, Earnest A., quoted, 77
Horace, quoted, 218
Hormones, 69–70, 73, 82, 180, 181
Human Body, The (Clendening), 51
Hydrocarbons, 117, 196
Hydrophile colloid, 191, 196
Hydrophobe colloid, 191, 196
Hypercholestremia, 115, 220, 221
Hypertension (high blood pressure),
    143
Hyperthyroidism, 146
Hypoadrenalism, 146
Hypoadrenia, 210, 211
Hysterectomy, 172

Ice cream, 193–96
Ichthyosis, 46
Immunizations, 39
Indians, American, 183, 189, 220
Indigestion, 111, 112, 116, 172, 190
Infant feeding, 109–12, 197–98, 209
Infarct, 139
Infectious diseases, 31, 39
Insanity, 128
Insulin, 122, 169, 170
Iodine, 58, 59, 117, 152
Iritis, 47

Jacobi, Abraham, 109
Johnson, Lyndon B., 165
Jones, Edith, 18
Journal of Laboratory and Clinical
    Medicine (Vaughan), 58
Journal of the American Dietetic
    Association, 228

Kidneys, 12, 42–43, 48, 123, 129–
    30, 182, 187, 196, 198, 220, 222

Lane, Sir W. Arbuthnot, 148–49
Latham, Peter Mere, 17
Laxatives, 148
Leucocytosis of childhood, 180
Leucopenia, 59, 180–81
Leukemia, 101, 189
Leveridge, Richard, quoted, 177
Life magazine, 26

Linneaus, Carl, *quoted*, 3
Liver, 6, 37, 42, 43, 45, 62–68, 83, 92, 93, 101, 123, 130, 136, 141, 145, 168, 172, 179, 180, 182, 183, 189, 192, 196, 197, 198, 205, 208, 210, 211, 216–17, 220
Los Angeles *Times*, 7, 18
Lungs, 42–43
Lymph glands, 104
Lymphocytes, 57–58, 59, 180–81
Lymphocytosis of childhood, 59

Mackenzie, Sir James, 126, 128, 223–24
MacMillan, Donald, 190
Man, the Unknown (Carrel), 153
Man and His Body (Miller and Goode), 62
Marriott, McKim, 121
Massachusetts Medical Society, 12–13
Mastoid disease, 47, 105
Mayo, William J., *quoted*, 14, 69
McCarrison, Sir Robert, *quoted*, 200
Measles, 103–04
Meat, 182, 188, 190, 191, 226, 227, 228
Medicine Today (Clark), 3
Medulla, 70
Meningitis, 47
Menopause, 173–74
Menstruation, 172–73, 274
Mesomorphs, 82
Metabolic water, 131–33, 136
Metabolism, 55, 72, 116, 187, 219
Migraine headache, 45–46, 205
Milk, 110–11, 179, 183–84, 188, 189, 197–98, 208–13
Milk diet, 210–11
Miller, Benjamin F., 62
Milton, John, *quoted*, 53
Mineral oil, 148
Minerals, 55, 56, 57, 60, 201, 203
Mitchell, P. H., 182
Mitchell, S. Weir, 96
Mitchell Textbook of General Physiology, 182
Molecules, 178, 191
Monopotassium glutamate, 147–48
Monosodium glutamate, 147–48
Morphine, 222, 223
Myxedema, 151

Natural foods, 282–83
"Natural water," 206
Nature, the greatest healer, xiv, 24, 30, 32, 36, 81, 109, 228; laws of, 34–35
Nephritis, 128
Nephrosis, 39, 205
Neuritis, 47
Nutrition, 218, 228; role of, 16–28
Nutritional science, xiii

Obesity, 51, 56–57, 143–54, 155–56; classification of, 149
Oils, 115, 203, 207
Organic salt, 165, 226, 227
Osler, Sir William, 10, 32, 49, 126, 165, 166, 168, 229
Our Synthetic Environment (Herber), 51–52
Overacidity, 187
Overweight, *see* Obesity
Oxidation, 47–48, 71, 120, 202–03

Pacific Northwest Indians, 189
Pain, 34
Pancreas, 205
Paré, Ambroise, 204
Paroxysmal tachycardia, 222
Pasteur, Louis, xiv, 33, 38, 39, 40, 41, 102
Pasteurization of milk, 110, 197, 212–13
Penicillin, 7, 259
Pericarditis, 47
Peritonitis, 47
Phenol, 207
Phlebitis, 239
Phosphorus, 146
Physical fitness, 4
Pimples, 106, 214
Pituitary gland, xv, 7, 8, 43, 45, 70, 72–74, 86, 90, 92, 96, 121
Pituitary-type body, 88–89, 95–96
Plagues, 33
Plains Indians, 183
Plato, 15, 31, 32
Plummer, R. H. A., 213
Pneumonia, 39
Polio, 101, 105, 113, 189, 195–96
Porter, Charles S., 210
Postgraduate Medicine (Holt), 187–88

Potassium, 204, 215
Pottenger, Francis F., Jr., 6, 191–92, 198, 213
Preventive medicine, 128
"Principles of Biological Oxidation" (Szent-Györgyi), 202–03
Prinzmetal, Myron, 125
Protein acids, 101, 104, 105
"Protein mania," 187–88
Proteins, 55, 57, 79, 208, 209, 226, 227, 228; as body builders, 177–85; as body killers, 186–99
Pseudo anginas, 121
Psoriasis, 46
Pustules, 106
Pyelitis, 47
Pyorrhea, 192

Ratner, Herbert, 158, 225–26; quoted, 29
Recent Advances in Chemistry in Relation to Medical Practice (Marriott), 121
Relation of Alimentation and Disease (Salisbury), 146
Research, medical, 4, 38
Rheumatism, 31, 101, 106–07, 133
Rice Diet, 149
Rockefeller, John D., Sr., 183
Root vegetables, 207
Rosenbaum, Francis F., 127
Roughage, 205, 226, 227
Rush, Benjamin, 219–20

St. Martin, Alexis, 57
Salisbury, James H., 57, 146, 147
Salt, 17, 25, 165, 166, 171, 219–22, 223, 224, 226; organic, 165, 226, 227
Sandler, Benjamin F., 195
Saturation, 116–18, 128, 147
Seborrhea capitus, 106
Selye, Hans, 34
Shakespeare, William, quoted, 54, 129
Shaw, George Bernard, 206
Sheldon, William H., 82, 89
Sherman, Henry C., 209
Sinusitis, 47
Skin diseases, 43, 46–47, 101, 147, 214

Small intestine, 56, 60, 65, 180, 193, 213, 228
Smallpox, 39, 107
Smith, Homer W., 131
Snively, William D., quoted, 62
Sodium, 37, 64–65, 204, 215, 217
Solar plexus, 59, 193
Somatotyping, 82
Somers, M. H. and A. R., 33
South Sea Islanders, 183
Spices, 207, 224
Spleen, 58, 181
Starches, 111, 146, 151, 173, 187, 196, 207, 226–27, 228
Starchy vegetables, 203, 206
Stefansson, Vilhjalmur, 116, 190, 227
Steroid drugs, 109
Stevenson, Ian, 30, 80
Stimulants, 109, 218–26
Stimulation, 182, 218–26
Stress of Life, The (Selye), 34
Stroke, 118
Strong Medicine (Donaldson), 148
Stomach, 180, 193, 209
Styes, 102, 106
Sugars, 60, 173, 187, 196, 207, 209, 226, 227, 228
Sulfas, 109
Surgery, 157–58, 159
Sweat glands, 133
Sweet vegetables, 203
Sydenham, Thomas, 12, 40, 49
Syndrome, 153
Syrus, Publius, 10
Szent-Györgyi, Albert V., 14–15, 125, 202–03

Taylor, Sir Henry, quoted, 186
Terramycin, 159
Thalidomide, 5, 59
Thompson, Furness, 4
Thomson, James C., 126–27, 213
Thoracic duct, 58
Thymus gland, 59, 181
Thyroid gland, xv, 6, 43, 45, 46–47, 57, 58, 59, 70, 72, 74, 75, 87, 89, 90, 92, 120, 122, 146, 148, 154, 163–64, 171, 181
Thyroid-type body, 86–88, 94–95, 155
Tilden, J. H., 49

Tobacco, 222, 224
Tongue, 210
Tonsillitis, 47, 101, 104-05, 198
Toxemia, 24, 43, 44, 51, 52, 92, 93,
  116, 168, 172, 174, 189, 194, 198,
  205, 227; of pregnancy, 5
Toxemia Explained (Tilden), 49
Toxic bloat, 145, 153-54
Toxic obesity, 149, 152-54
Toxins, xiv, 42, 45, 65, 74, 108, 111,
  128, 172, 173, 217; elimination of,
  4-5, 42-49, 174
Tranquilizers, 6
Tuberculosis, 31, 102, 146, 172
Tubular disease, 138
Tumors, 21-23, 84, 115, 227
Twain, Mark, 144
Typhoid fever, 39

Ulcers, 37, 66, 200-01, 214
"Undulant" fever, 212
Underweight, problem of, 154-55
U.S. Commission on Chronic Ill-
  nesses, 52

Vaughan, Warren T., 58
Vegetable juices, raw, 206, 229
Vegetables, 200-07, 227
Vegetarianism, 206
Villi, 56, 60
Virchow, Rudolf, 33
Viruses, 31
Vis medicatrix naturae, 41
Vitamins, 9, 55, 60, 179, 197, 203,
  204, 206, 207, 213, 214, 215, 217,
  226, 227
Volney, Constantin, 27

Water, 131-33, 136, 206, 226
Weger, George S., 49
Weight problems, *see* Obesity; Un-
  derweight
Williams, Leonard, 210
Women's ailments, 172-74

Yeast, 37, 213-17
Young, Brigham, 204

About the Author

DR. HENRY G. BIELER studied medicine at the University of Cincinnati, where he came under the life-long influence of Dr. Martin Fischer, the great physiologist and philosopher. For over fifty years he was a doctor and treated great motion-picture stars, coal miners, politicians and professional men, farmers and Pasadena dowagers. He brought thousands of healthy babies into the world, including his own children and grandchildren. He died in October 1975.